W9-AYC-716

Essential Drug Dosage Calculations

THIRD EDITION

Lorrie N. Hegstad, RN, PhD
Associate Professor
School of Nursing
The University of Texas at Arlington
Arlington, Texas

Wilma Hayek, RN, MSN
Assistant Professor
School of Nursing
The University of Texas Health Science Center at San Antonio
San Antonio, Texas

APPLETON & LANGE
Norwalk, Connecticut

Copyright © 1994 by Appleton & Lange
Simon & Schuster Business and Professional Group
Copyright © 1989 by Appleton & Lange
Copyright © 1983 by Robert J. Brady Company

94 95 96 97 98 / 10 9 8 7 6 5 4 3 2

Prentice Hall International (UK) Limited, *London*
Prentice Hall of Australia Pty. Limited, *Sydney*
Prentice Hall Canada, Inc., *Toronto*
Prentice Hall Hispanoamericana, S.A., *Mexico*
Prentice Hall of India Private Limited, *New Delhi*
Prentice Hall of Japan, Inc., *Tokyo*
Simon & Schuster Asia Pte. Ltd., *Singapore*
Editora Prentice Hall do Brasil Ltda., *Rio de Janeiro*
Prentice Hall, *Englewood Cliffs, New Jersey*

Library of Congress Cataloging-in-Publication Data

Hegstad, Lorrie N., 1945–
    Essential drug dosage calculations / Lorrie N. Hegstad, Wilma
Hayek.—3rd ed.
        p. cm.
    ISBN 0-8385-2038-3
    1. Pharmaceutical arithmetic. 2. Nursing—Mathematics.
I. Hayek, Wilma, 1939–   . II. Title.
    [DNLM: 1. Drugs—administration & dosage. 2. Mathematics.   QV 748
H464e   1993]
RS57.H44   1993
615′.14—dc20
DNLM/DLC
for Library of Congress   93-8445
                                          CIP

Acquisitions Editor: Sally J. Barhydt
Production Editor: Karen Davis
Designer: Penny Kindzierski
Interior Art: Kathleen D. Hornyak

ISBN 0-8385-2038-3

9 780838 520383

90000

Contents

Preface

The purpose of this book is to assist the learner in developing competence in the interpretation of medication orders and the calculation of correct dosages. It is written primarily for students enrolled in professional and technical schools of nursing. However, it can also serve as a reference for practicing nurses or as a part of in-service education refresher courses for inactive nurses. The book can be used as a self-paced independent learning module or within a planned course. Illustrations of measuring devices and drug forms are provided to aid the learner's understanding of the content.

Essential Drug Dosage Calculations presents the proportion method as a simple and practical approach to the calculating of dosages and solutions. Both generic and trade names of drugs are used throughout the text to help the learner become familiar with the current dosage forms and quantities.

The third edition of *Essential Drug Dosage Calculations* has expanded on topics in several areas to keep up with changes in medications and administration. Significant changes in the third edition include the following:

- New section on interpreting drug labels to prepare and administer drugs

- Over 50 different drug labels used in problems throughout the text

- Inclusion of only frequently used and new drugs

- Additional practice problems in each chapter, over 500 in all

- Major revision of the insulin and the intravenous fluids and medications chapters

- Additional comprehensive test questions

Each chapter introduces the type of problem with a step-by-step procedure for straightforward solution. Simple and complex examples are included, followed by a wide range of practice problems. To provide immediate feedback and to aid in reinforcing learning, each problem is set up in the appropriate proportion or formula and solved. Two comprehensive exams round out the edition to provide the learner with additional practice and an opportunity to experience test-taking.

Every effort has been made to make this third edition an even more successful learning tool for students and to help them master critical knowledge so basic to their careers in nursing.

Acknowledgments

We wish to thank the many nursing and health care educators who adopted our book and returned evaluations. The comments provided us direction for the changes made in the third edition. We also wish to express our appreciation to the students in schools of nursing who have used this book and provided us with feedback.

Our appreciation goes to faculty at The University of Texas at Arlington, Susan Chappell, MSN, RN, CDE, for her review of the insulin chapter, and Susan Pixler, MSN, RN, PNP, for review of calculating dosages for infants and children. We would also like to thank the staff at Appleton & Lange for their continued support.

Lorrie N. Hegstad
Wilma Hayek

Objectives

Upon completion of this book, the learner should be able to:

1. Identify abbreviations and symbols used in the preparation and administration of medications.
2. Interpret medication orders and drug labels.
3. Identify units of measure appropriate to the household, metric, and apothecary systems.
4. Derive the approximate equivalent, convert from one system of measurement to another or from one unit of measurement to another within the same system.
5. Calculate the correct oral dosage in tablet or liquid form to be administered to the patient.
6. Given a parenteral drug in liquid form, calculate the correct volume to be administered to equal the dosage ordered.
7. Given a parenteral drug in its dry form, determine the correct:
   a. vial of medication to reconstitute
   b. amount of diluent to add to obtain the prescribed dosage
   c. total reconstituted volume
   d. volume of displacement
   e. volume of drug to administer to equal the prescribed dosage.
8. Label the reconstituted parenteral drug with the specific dosage for volume and the discard date.
9. Given a patient's weight in pounds or kilograms, determine a safe dose.
10. Given U-100 insulin and a U-100/1 cc, U-100/0.5 cc, U-100/0.3 cc, or U-100/0.25 cc syringe, identify the quantity of insulin to be administered to equal the prescribed dosage.
11. Using U-100 insulin and a tuberculin syringe, compute the correct volume of insulin to be administered to equal the prescribed dosage.
12. Given a sliding scale prescribed by a physician and the blood sugar results of the patient, compute the correct volume of insulin to be administered.
13. Given a specific IV administration set and the volume of solution to infuse per hour(s), calculate the correct:
   a. drop rate per minute

     b. length of time needed to infuse the total amount ordered

     c. total volume of fluid infused over a specified period of time.

14. Determine the IV drop rate needed to deliver a specified dosage of a medication in a limited period of time.

15. Given a prescribed dose of medication to be administered IV push, determine the:

     a. amount of diluent to add to the medication

     b. volume of diluted drug to be administered in a specific time period.

16. Calculate the body surface area of a child, using the nomogram.

17. Calculate the safe pediatric dose using body weight and the body surface formula.

Basic Arithmetic

Basic Arithmetic Pretest

Write the following roman numerals in arabic numbers:

1. v _____   2. ss _____

3. iii _____   4. i _____

5. x _____   6. xv _____

7. vii _____   8. xx _____

Write the following arabic numbers in roman numerals:

9. 2 _____   10. 1½ _____

11. 5 _____   12. 8 _____

13. 12 _____   14. 4 _____

15. 6 _____   16. 9 _____

Solve the following to the lowest possible fraction or two decimal places:

Fractions

17. $\frac{1}{4} + \frac{2}{4} =$ 18. $\frac{1}{10} + \frac{3}{5} =$

19. $\frac{1}{150} + \frac{1}{300} =$ 20. $\frac{2}{7} + \frac{1}{3} =$

21. $\frac{4}{5} - \frac{1}{5} =$ 22. $\frac{3}{4} - \frac{1}{3} =$

23. $\frac{1}{100} - \frac{1}{150} =$ 24. $\frac{4}{6} - \frac{3}{8} =$

25. $\frac{2}{3} \times \frac{4}{5}$ =

26. $\frac{1}{10} \times \frac{1}{6}$ =

27. $\frac{1}{100} \times \frac{1}{5}$ =

28. $\frac{3}{8} \times \frac{5}{6}$ =

29. $\frac{1}{8} \div \frac{1}{64}$ =

30. $\frac{1}{6} \div 6$ =

31. $\frac{1}{150} \div \frac{1}{2}$ =

32. $\frac{3}{5} \div \frac{3}{9}$ =

Decimals

33. $1.5 + 1.3$ =

34. $0.32 + 1.9$ =

35. $23.67 + 4.30$ =

36. $0.05 + 0.004$ =

37. $0.06 - 0.02$ =

38. $8 - 0.87$ =

39. $4.32 - 0.013$ =

40. $1.37 - 0.26$ =

41. 2.36×0.002 =

42. 1.06×1.13 =

43. 0.006×4.3 =

44. 0.25×100 =

45. $0.06 \div 0.02$ =

46. $1.50 \div 0.30$ =

47. $7.5 \div 0.035$ =

48. $26.45 \div 3.60$ =

Conversions: Convert the term given to its correct *percentage, fraction,* or *decimal* value. One value is given; calculate the other two equivalent values.

Percent	Common Fraction	Decimal
49. ____	$\frac{1}{2}$	50. ____
25%	51. ____	52. ____
53. ____	54. ____	0.10
0.9%	55. ____	56. ____
57. ____	$\frac{1}{3}$	58. ____
59. ____	60. ____	0.001

Find the value of X in these proportion-type problems:

61. $3 : X :: 2 : 12$ =

62. $X : 6 :: 4 : 3$ =

63. $\frac{1}{4} : X :: 1 : 8 =$

64. $48 : 12 :: \frac{1}{10} : X =$

65. $\frac{2}{3} : \frac{3}{5} :: X : \frac{9}{10} =$

66. $\frac{1}{2} : X :: 0.125 : 4 =$

67. $0.25 : 500 :: X : 1000 =$

68. $\frac{4}{5} : 50 :: X : 100 =$

69. $\frac{1}{150} : \frac{1}{200} :: 4 : X =$

70. $X : 12 :: 1.5 : 60 =$

Solve the following word problems:

71. A student gets 3 credits for each course. If the student has a total of 30 credits, how many courses has the student taken?

72. If there are 2 ounces of a drug in 32 ounces of a solution, how many ounces of the drug are there in 16 ounces of the same solution?

73. Your salary is $125.00 per week. You plan to place at least 10% each week in savings. How much would you save each month (4 weeks)?

74. If one tablet contains gr (grain) $\frac{1}{100}$ of a drug, how many grains would be in 3 tablets?

75. The doctor ordered 40 milligrams of a drug. The label on the bottle says that each tablet contains 5 milligrams. How many tablets are needed to equal the doctor's order?

☐ Answers

Roman numerals in arabic numbers:

1. 5	2. $\frac{1}{2}$	3. 3	4. 1
5. 10	6. 15	7. 7	8. 20

Arabic numbers in roman numerals:

9. ii	10. iss	11. v	12. viii
13. xii	14. iv	15. vi	16. ix

Fractions

17. ¾	18. $\frac{7}{10}$	19. $\frac{1}{100}$
20. $\frac{13}{21}$	21. ⅗	22. $\frac{5}{12}$
23. $\frac{1}{300}$	24. $\frac{7}{24}$	25. $\frac{8}{15}$
26. $\frac{1}{60}$	27. $\frac{1}{500}$	28. $\frac{5}{16}$
29. 8	30. $\frac{1}{36}$	31. $\frac{1}{75}$
32. 1⅘		

Decimals

33. 2.8	34. 2.22	35. 27.97
36. 0.054	37. 0.04	38. 7.13
39. 4.307	40. 1.11	41. 0.00472
42. 1.1978	43. 0.0258	44. 25
45. 3	46. 5	47. 214.2857
48. 7.347		

Conversions:

49. 50%	50. 0.50
51. ¼	52. 0.25
53. 10%	54. $\frac{1}{10}$
55. $\frac{9}{1000}$	56. 0.009
57. 33⅓%	58. 0.333
59. 0.1%	60. $\frac{1}{1000}$

Value of X:		Word problems:
61. 18	62. 8	71. 10 courses
63. 2	64. $\frac{1}{40}$	72. 1 ounce
65. 1	66. 16	73. $50.00 per month
67. 0.5	68. 1.6	74. $\frac{3}{100}$ grains
69. 3	70. 0.3	75. 8 tablets

Note to the Learner:
   This test contained the basic math skills needed to compute most dosage and solution problems. If you incorrectly answered more than three problems in each of the first sections or more than one of the word problems, you might find it helpful to complete the Review of Basic Arithmetic section before continuing the book.

Fractions

Definition: A fraction is a part of a whole.

$$\frac{4}{6} \frac{\text{NUMERATOR}}{\text{DENOMINATOR}}$$

Adding Fractions with Like Denominators

1. Add the numerators.

2. Place the answer over the denominator.

3. Reduce the answer to the lowest term by dividing the numerator and the denominator by the largest number that can divide them both.

Example

  a. 1. $\dfrac{1}{4} + \dfrac{1}{4} = \dfrac{1+1}{4} = \dfrac{2}{4}$

      2. $\dfrac{2}{4}\!\!>$ 2 is divisible into both numbers

      3. $\dfrac{\overset{1}{\cancel{2}}}{\underset{2}{\cancel{4}}} = \dfrac{1}{2}$

  b. 1. $\dfrac{3}{6} + \dfrac{3}{6} = \dfrac{3+3}{6} = \dfrac{6}{6}$

      2. $\dfrac{6}{6}\!\!>$ 6 is divisible into both numbers

      3. $\dfrac{\overset{1}{\cancel{6}}}{\underset{1}{\cancel{6}}} = 1$

Adding Fractions with Unlike Denominators

1. Find the smallest number that the denominators of each fraction divide into evenly (least common denominator).

2. Divide the denominator into the least common denominator and multiply the results by the numerator.

3. Add the new numerators and place over the new denominator (least common denominator).

4. Reduce to lowest terms.

Example

   a. 1. $\dfrac{1}{4} + \dfrac{1}{3}$ (4 and 3 will divide into 12 evenly)

     2. $12 \div 4 = 3 \times 1 = 3$

        $12 \div 3 = 4 \times 1 = 4$

     3. $\dfrac{3 + 4}{12}$

     4. $\dfrac{7}{12}$ is reduced to lowest terms

   b. 1. $\dfrac{1}{6} + \dfrac{1}{2}$ (6 and 2 will divide into 6 evenly)

     2. $6 \div 6 = 1 \times 1 = 1$

        $6 \div 2 = 3 \times 1 = 3$

     3. $\dfrac{1 + 3}{6}$

     4. $\dfrac{\overset{2}{\cancel{4}}}{\underset{3}{\cancel{6}}}$ > both numbers evenly divided by 2

       $\frac{2}{3}$ is reduced to lowest terms

Subtracting Fractions with Like Denominators

1. Subtract the numerators.

2. Place the difference over the denominator.

3. Reduce to lowest terms.

Example

   a. 1. $\dfrac{3}{4} - \dfrac{1}{4} = \dfrac{3 - 1}{4}$

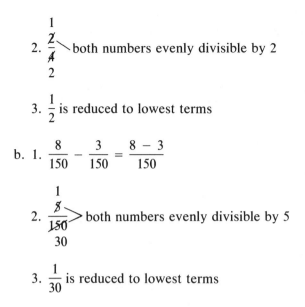

2. $\dfrac{\cancel{2}^{1}}{\cancel{4}^{2}}$ ⟍ both numbers evenly divisible by 2

3. $\dfrac{1}{2}$ is reduced to lowest terms

b. 1. $\dfrac{8}{150} - \dfrac{3}{150} = \dfrac{8-3}{150}$

2. $\dfrac{\cancel{5}^{1}}{\cancel{150}_{30}}$ ⟩ both numbers evenly divisible by 5

3. $\dfrac{1}{30}$ is reduced to lowest terms

Subtracting Fractions with Unlike Denominators

1. Find the least common denominator and convert fractions.

2. Subtract the numerators.

3. Place the difference over the least common denominator.

4. Reduce to lowest terms.

Example

a. 1. $\dfrac{3}{2} - \dfrac{3}{4}$ (both 2 and 4 divisible into 4)

   $4 \div 2 = 2 \times 3 = 6$

   $4 \div 4 = 1 \times 3 = 3$

2. $\dfrac{6}{4} - \dfrac{3}{4} = \dfrac{6-3}{4}$

3. $\dfrac{3}{4}$

4. $\dfrac{3}{4}$ is reduced to lowest terms

b. 1. $\dfrac{1}{100} - \dfrac{1}{150}$ (both 100 and 150 divisible into 300)

$300 \div 100 = 3 \times 1 = 3$

$300 \div 150 = 2 \times 1 = 2$

2. $\dfrac{3}{300} - \dfrac{2}{300} = \dfrac{3-2}{300}$

3. $\dfrac{1}{300}$

4. $\dfrac{1}{300}$ is reduced to lowest terms

Multiplying Fractions

1. Multiply the numerators.

2. Multiply the denominators.

3. Reduce to lowest terms.

Example

a. 1. & 2. $\dfrac{2}{3} \times \dfrac{3}{4} = \dfrac{2 \times 3}{3 \times 4} = \dfrac{6}{12}$ (6 will divide evenly into 6 and 12)

3. $\dfrac{\overset{1}{\cancel{6}}}{\underset{2}{\cancel{12}}} = \dfrac{1}{2}$ (reduced to lowest terms)

b. 1. & 2. $\dfrac{1}{8} \times \dfrac{4}{9} = \dfrac{1 \times 4}{8 \times 9} = \dfrac{4}{72}$ (4 will divide evenly into both numbers)

3. $\dfrac{\overset{1}{\cancel{4}}}{\underset{18}{\cancel{72}}} = \dfrac{1}{18}$ (reduced to lowest terms)

c. 1. & 2. $\dfrac{1}{100} \times \dfrac{1}{3} = \dfrac{1 \times 1}{100 \times 3} = \dfrac{1}{300}$

3. $\dfrac{1}{300}$ is reduced to lowest terms

Dividing Fractions

1. Invert the divisor $\left(\frac{1}{2} \text{ would become } \frac{2}{1}\right)$.

2. Change the divison sign ($\div$) to multiplication ($\times$).

3. Multiply the numerators.

4. Multiply the denominators.

5. Reduce to lowest terms.

$$
\begin{array}{cc}
\text{Dividend} & \text{Divisor} \\
\frac{1}{4} \quad \div & \frac{1}{2}
\end{array}
$$

Example

a. $\dfrac{1}{4} \div \dfrac{1}{2} = \dfrac{1}{4} \times \dfrac{2}{1} = \dfrac{1 \times 2}{4 \times 1} = \dfrac{2}{4} = \dfrac{1}{2}$

b. $\dfrac{1}{2} \div 100 = \dfrac{1}{2} \times \dfrac{1}{100} = \dfrac{1 \times 1}{2 \times 100} = \dfrac{1}{200}$

c. $\dfrac{1}{150} \div \dfrac{1}{300} = \dfrac{1}{150} \times \dfrac{300}{1} = \dfrac{300}{150} = 2$

Decimals

Definition: A fraction whose denominator is a power of 10 expressed by placing a point at the left of the numerator.

Example

$$\frac{2}{10} = 0.2 \qquad \frac{25}{100} = 0.25$$

To CHANGE *fractions to decimals,* divide the numerator by the denominator.

Example

a. $\dfrac{1}{4} = 4\overline{)\begin{array}{r} 0.25 \\ 1.00 \end{array}}$

$$\begin{array}{r} \underline{0} \\ 10 \\ \underline{8} \\ 20 \\ \underline{20} \end{array}$$

b. $\dfrac{2}{3} = 3\overline{)\begin{array}{r} 0.666 \text{ or } 0.67 \\ 2.00 \end{array}}$

$$\begin{array}{r} \underline{0} \\ 20 \\ \underline{18} \\ 20 \\ \underline{18} \\ 20 \\ \underline{18} \\ 2 \end{array}$$

c. $\dfrac{1}{150} = 150\overline{)\begin{array}{r} 0.0066 \\ 1.000 \end{array}}$

$$\begin{array}{r} \underline{0} \\ 10 \\ \underline{00} \\ 100 \\ \underline{000} \\ 1000 \\ \underline{900} \\ 1000 \\ \underline{900} \\ 100 \end{array}$$

Adding Decimals

Align the decimals and add.

Example

$$\begin{array}{r} 1.36 \\ 1.20 \\ 0.05 \\ \underline{4.60} \\ 7.21 \end{array}$$

Subtracting Decimals

Align the decimals and subtract.

Example

a.   1.36
   − 0.04
   _____
     1.32

b.   4.00
   − 1.39
   _____
     2.61

Multiplying Decimals

1. Multiply as whole numbers.

2. Count the number of decimal places in the multiplier and the multiplicand.

3. Count from right to left in the product and place the decimal point.

Example

a.   1.56 multiplicand
   × 0.34 multiplier
   _____
      624
     468
    000
   _____
   0.5304 product (4 decimal places)

b.   0.36
   × 0.4
   _____
      144
    000
   _____
   0.144 (3 decimal places)

Dividing Decimals

1. Convert the divisor to a whole number by moving the decimal point to the right.

2. Move the decimal point in the dividend the *same* number of places to the right as in the divisor.

3. Divide as usual.

4. Place the decimal point in the answer (quotient) directly above the decimal point in the dividend.

5. Carry out the answer to 3 decimal places before rounding off to 2 places.

Example

$$\text{a. } 36 \div 1.2 = \text{(divisor) } 1.2\overline{)36.0000} \text{ (dividend)}$$

$$\begin{array}{r} 30.000 \text{ (quotient)} \\ \underline{36} \\ 0 \\ \underline{0} \end{array}$$

$$\text{b. } 1.25 \div 0.75 = 0.75\overline{)1.25000}$$

$$\begin{array}{r} 1.666 \text{ or } 1.67 \\ \underline{75} \\ 500 \\ \underline{450} \\ 500 \\ \underline{450} \end{array}$$

Percentage

Definition: A percentage is a part of 100.

To CHANGE percent to common fraction, place the percent in the numerator with 100 as the denominator.

Example

$$\text{a. } 10\% = \frac{10}{100} = 10 \div 100 = \frac{1}{10}$$

$$\text{b. } \frac{1}{4}\% = \frac{\frac{1}{4}}{100} = \frac{1}{4} \div \frac{100^*}{1} = \frac{1}{4} \times \frac{1}{100^*} = \frac{1}{400}$$

$$\text{c. } 0.9\% = \frac{\frac{9}{10}}{100} = \frac{9}{10} \div \frac{100}{1} = \frac{9}{10} \times \frac{1}{100} = \frac{9}{1000}$$

To CHANGE common fractions to percents divide the numerator by the

---

* Remember to invert the divisor and then multiply.

denominator and multiply the quotient by 100 (or move the decimal point 2 places to the right).

Example

a. $\dfrac{1}{4} =$
$$\begin{array}{r} 0.25 \\ 4\,\overline{)1.000} \\ \underline{8} \\ 20 \\ \underline{20} \\ 00 \end{array}$$
$$\begin{array}{r} 0.25 \\ \times\ 100 \\ \hline 25.00 \text{ or } 25\% \end{array}$$

b. $\dfrac{1}{100} =$
$$\begin{array}{r} 0.01 \\ 100\,\overline{)1.000} \\ \underline{0} \\ 10 \\ \underline{0} \\ 100 \\ \underline{100} \end{array}$$
$$\begin{array}{r} 0.01 \\ \times\ 100 \\ \hline 1.00 \text{ or } 1\% \end{array}$$

To CHANGE percent to decimal fraction remove the % sign and divide by 100 (move the decimal point two places to the left).

Example

a. 10% = 0.10
$$\begin{array}{r} 0.10 \\ 100\,\overline{)10.00} \\ \underline{0} \\ 100 \\ \underline{100} \end{array}$$

b. 0.1% = 0.001
$$\begin{array}{r} 0.001 \\ 100\,\overline{)0.1000} \\ \underline{0} \\ 1 \\ \underline{0} \\ 10 \\ \underline{0} \\ 100 \\ \underline{100} \end{array}$$

Ratio and Proportion

Definition: Ratio is composed of two numbers that share a distinct relationship. They are separated by a colon (:).

Example   4 : 8 or 50 : 1

Definition: A proportion consists of two ratios that have the same value.

Example   5 : 20 :: 2 : 8

In solving ratio and proportion problems one of the numbers is "unknown."

Example

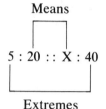

Means

5 : 20 :: X : 40

Extremes

The two center numbers are known as the means and the two outer numbers are known as the extremes. The "X" may be in any of the four positions.

To solve for the "unknown" or "X"

1. Multiply the means.

2. Multiply the extremes.

3. Place the product with the "X" to the left of the equals mark and solve the equation by dividing the entire equation by the number before the "X."

4. To prove that your answer is correct, substitute the answer for the X in the problem, multiply the means (inside numbers), and then multiply the extremes (outside numbers). The numbers should be the same.

Example

a. 5 : 20 :: 2 : X   Proof:

$$5X = 40$$

$$\frac{5X}{5} = \frac{40}{5}$$

$$X = 8$$

40

5 : 20 :: 2 : 8

40

b.
$$X : \frac{1}{150} :: 1 : \frac{1}{100}$$

$$\frac{1}{100} X = \frac{1}{150}$$

$$\frac{\frac{1}{100}}{\frac{1}{100}} X = \frac{\frac{1}{150}}{\frac{1}{100}}$$

$$X = \frac{1}{150} \div \frac{1}{100} = \frac{1}{150} \times \frac{100}{1} = \frac{100}{150} = \frac{2}{3}$$

Proof:

$$\frac{2}{3} : \frac{1}{150} :: 1 : \frac{1}{100}$$

$$\frac{2}{300} \text{ or } \frac{1}{150}$$

The use of ratio and proportion to set up and solve dosage and solution problems will be discussed in greater detail later.

Metric System of Measurement

The metric system of weights and measures is used extensively in the medical and scientific community. It is the system of choice when dealing with drug dosages, owing to the accuracy and simplicity of the system. The metric system is a decimal system (base 10), and the math needed to work within the system is accomplished by moving the decimal to the right or left.

Only a few of the many metric weights and measures are commonly used in the preparation of medications (Table 2.1). The most common units are gram (Gm, g, gm); milligram (mg); microgram (μg); kilogram (kg); milliliter (mL, ml, mℓ); cubic centimeter (cc); and liter (L).

TABLE 2.1. Metric Equivalents[a]

Volume

1 liter = 1000 mL (milliliters) or cc (cubic centimeters)
Note: milliliter and cubic centimeter are used interchangeably.

Weight

1 mg (milligram)	=	1000 μg[b] (microgram)
1 Gm (gram)	=	1000 mg (milligrams)
1 kg (kilogram)[c]	=	1000 Gm (grams)

[a] An equivalent is a unit of measure that is considered to be of equal or approximate value to a unit of measure expressed in the same system or in a different system of measurement.
[b] μg is the International Systems of Units (SI) for microgram and should be used instead of mcg. Because the manufacturers of drugs and some drug references continue to use mcg, it will be used on occasion throughout the text.
[c] 1 kg = 2.2 lbs. The avoirdupois pound (16 ounces = 1 pound) is used as the equivalent in calculating drugs according to body weight.

The following rules will be very helpful when you use the metric system:

Metric System Rules

1. Arabic numbers are used: 1; 5; 100.

2. Quantities less than 1 are always expressed as decimal fractions: 0.2; 0.008; 1.5; 46.03.

3. To emphasize the decimal point, place a *zero* in front of the decimal not preceded by a whole number: 0.05; 0.001.

4. When metric abbreviations are used, the arabic numeral precedes the abbreviation: 20 Gm; 50 mL; 1000 mg; 1.5 cc.

5. The abbreviation for gram (Gm) should be capitalized to distinguish it from grain (gr). This is especially important when the abbreviation is handwritten. If gr (grain) is not written carefully it could be mistaken for gm (gram). Some drug companies use the abbreviation g or gm for gram, and careful reading is required to distinguish it from gr (grain).

6. To convert

> liters   to milliliters
>
> grams   to milligrams
>
> milligrams to micrograms
>
> kilograms to grams

multiply by 1000 or move the decimal point 3 places to the right.

Example

  1 liter   = 1000 milliliters

  1.1 gram   = 1100 milligrams

  5 milligrams = 5000 micrograms

  2 kilograms   = 2000 grams

7. To convert

> milliliters   to liters
>
> milligrams   to grams
>
> micrograms to milligrams
>
> grams   to kilograms

divide by 1000 or move the decimal point 3 places to the left.

Example

  500 milliliters   = 0.5 liters

  1500 milligrams   = 1.5 grams

  10,000 micrograms = 10 milligrams

  4500 grams   = 4.5 kilograms

Complete the Practice Problems to test your knowledge of metric equivalents by using the conversion methods defined in numbers 6 and 7.

☐ Practice Problems

Directions
Change each item to the appropriate equivalent.

1. 1 Gm = _____ mg		2. 750 mg = _____ Gm
3. 500 mL = _____ liter		4. 0.060 Gm = _____ mg
5. 350 mg = _____ μg		6. 0.5 g = _____ mg
7. 100 mg = _____ Gm		8. 2500 Gm = _____ kg
9. 0.25 Gm = _____ mg		10. 4.5 liters = _____ mL
11. 10 mg = _____ Gm		12. 30 kg = _____ Gm
13. 1500 μg = _____ mg		14. 0.001 Gm = _____ mg
15. 1 liter = _____ mL		16. 4 μg = _____ mg
17. 1.1 g = _____ mg		18. 50 mL = _____ liter
19. 2 mg = _____ Gm		20. 0.125 mg = _____ μg
21. 280 mL = _____ liter		22. 1780 Gm = _____ kg
23. 2.4 Gm = _____ mg		24. 3 mg = _____ μg
25. 0.69 liter = _____ mL		26. 55.5 mg = _____ Gm
27. 75 mcg = _____ mg		28. 1 kg = _____ g
29. 440 mL = _____ liter		30. 3000 mg = _____ Gm

☐ **Answers**

1. 1000 mg	2. 0.750 Gm
3. 0.5 liter	4. 60 mg
5. 350,000 μg	6. 500 mg
7. 0.1 Gm	8. 2.5 kg
9. 250 mg	10. 4500 mL
11. 0.010 Gm	12. 30,000 Gm
13. 1.5 mg	14. 1 mg
15. 1000 mL	16. 0.004 mg
17. 1100 mg	18. 0.05 liter
19. 0.002 Gm	20. 125 μg
21. 0.28 liter	22. 1.78 kg
23. 2400 mg	24. 3000 μg
25. 690 mL	26. 0.0555 Gm
27. 0.075 mg	28. 1000 g
29. 0.44 liter	30. 3 Gm

If you missed more than three of the problems, you should review the chapter before going to the next section.

Apothecaries' and Household Systems of Measurement

Apothecaries' System

The apothecaries' system of weights and measures (Table 3.1) was brought to the United States from England. Although the current government policy is aimed at converting to the metric system, this has not been totally achieved. Knowledge of all systems will be necessary for several years in order to administer medications accurately and safely.

TABLE 3.1. Apothecaries' Equivalents

Volume		
60 minims	=	1 fluid dram (ʒ i)*
4 drams (ʒ iv)	=	½ ounce (℥ ss)
8 drams (ʒ viii)	=	1 ounce (℥ i)
16 ounces (℥ xvi)	=	1 pint (pt)
32 ounces (℥ xxxii)	=	1 quart (qt)
2 pints	=	1 quart
4 quarts	=	1 gallon
Weight[a]		
60 grains (gr 1x)	=	1 dram (ʒ i)
8 drams (ʒ viii)	=	1 ounce (℥ i)
12 ounces (℥ xii)	=	1 pound

* When ounces or drams are used in medication orders or on drug labels, the word *fluid* is omitted and the order refers to unit of volume, not unit of weight.

[a] The dram and ounce, as units of weight, are rarely used by nurses to compute dosages. An avoirdupois pound (16 ounces = 1 pound) is more common than an apothecaries' pound (12 ounces = 1 pound).

Units of weight and units of volume are used in calculating correct dosages. The most commonly used units are:

Weight	*Volume*
Grain	Minim
	Dram
	Ounce
	Pint
	Quart

The apothecaries' system has special symbols and abbreviations associated with the specific units:

Unit	*Abbreviation or Symbol*
Grain	gr
Minim	m; min; ♏
Dram	dr; ʒ
Ounce	oz; ʒ
Pint	pt
Quart	qt

When using the apothecaries' system it is important to remember the following rules:

APOTHECARIES' RULES

1. Roman numerals are used to express numbers, such as vi for 6, x for 10, and xiv for 14.

2. When the numeral 1 (one) is used, a dot is placed over it to avoid confusion with the Roman numeral L (50): gr i; gr xi; gr viii.

3. When apothecary abbreviations are used, the numerals are written after the abbreviations: gr vii; ʒ x; ʒ xiv; ♏ xii.

4. Quantities less than 1 (one) are expressed as common fractions: gr ¼; gr ⅓.

5. The fraction not expressed as a common fraction is ½, which is written as ss: gr ss (grain ½); gr iss (grain 1½); gr viiss (grain 7½).

6. If abbreviations are not used, the numeral is expressed as an arabic number and precedes the designated unit: 6 grains, 3½ ounces; 4 drams.

Household System

The household system of measurement (Table 3.2) is used infrequently in the hospital. Because most household measuring devices lack standardization in their manufacture, they are not safe for measuring drugs. Household

TABLE 3.2. Commonly Used Household Measures

Household		Apothecary
1 teaspoon (tsp or t)	=	1 dram
1 teaspoon (tsp or t)	=	60 drops (gtts)[a]
3 teaspoons	=	½ ounce
1 tablespoon (tbsp or T)	=	½ ounce
2 tablespoons	=	1 ounce
Teacup	=	6 ounces
Glass or cup	=	8 ounces

Note: These equivalents are considered standard *but* remember they are only approximations.
[a] The size of a drop is dependent on many factors; the dropper size, the angle at which the dropper is held, and the type or viscosity of the liquid being dispensed. The drop equivalent should not be used indiscriminately. Most medications have special calibrated droppers, which should be used in preparing the drug.

measures should not be used when other measures are available. On occasion it may be necessary to determine approximate equivalents between the household, the apothecaries', and the metric system of measure; thus the nurse should be familiar with the most commonly used household measures.

☐ Practice Problems

Directions
Complete the practice problems to test your knowledge of the apothecary and household equivalents by using the tables provided.

1. ℥ i = _____ tbsp

2. 1 qt = _____ pts

3. 1 tbsp = _____ tsp

4. 1 ounce = _____ ʒ

5. 1 cup = _____ ounces

6. ʒ i = _____ minims

7. ℥ ss = _____ dram

8. 2 tbsp = _____ oz

9. 3 tsp = _____ oz

10. 1 pt = _____ ℥

11. 60 minims = _____ dram

12. ʒ i = _____ tsp

13. 1 teacup = _____ ounces

14. ℥ ss = _____ tsp

15. 32 ounces = _____ qt

16. 1 tbsp = _____ ounce

17. ʒ viii = _____ ℥

18. 60 grains = _____ dram

19. 1 gallon = _____ quarts

20. 8 ounces = _____ glass

21. 3 tsp = _____ tbsp

22. 1 qt = _____ ounces

23. 1 tsp = _____ dram

24. ℥ viii = _____ cup

25. ℥ iv = _____ ℥

26. 6 oz = _____ teacup

27. 16 oz = _____ pt

28. ℥ ss = _____ tbsp

29. 2 pts = _____ qt

30. 1 dram = _____ gr

☐ **Answers**

1. 2 tablespoons
2. 2 pints
3. 3 teaspoons
4. 8 drams
5. 8 ounces
6. 60 minims
7. 4 drams
8. 1 ounce
9. ½ ounce
10. 16 ounces
11. 1 dram
12. 1 teaspoon
13. 6 ounces
14. 3 teaspoons
15. 1 quart
16. ½ ounce
17. 1 ounce
18. 1 dram
19. 4 quarts
20. 1 glass
21. 1 tablespoon
22. 32 ounces
23. 1 dram
24. 1 cup
25. ½ ounce
26. 1 teacup
27. 1 pint
28. 1 tablespoon
29. 1 quart
30. 60 grains

If you missed more than three equivalents, you might wish to review the tables before going to the next section.

Interpretation of Medication Orders and Labels

The correct interpretation of the medication order and the medication label is the responsibility of the individual preparing the medication for administration. A variety of abbreviations and symbols is used in writing the medication order. It is the responsibility of the nurse to know the common abbreviations and symbols so the medication order can be interpreted correctly. The following abbreviations and symbols are essential for accurate interpretation of medication orders and the labels on medication containers.

Abbreviations and Symbols

aa; $\overline{aa}$	of each
a.c.; ac	before meals
A.D.	right ear
ad lib	as desired
A.L. or A.S.	left ear
A.M.; a.m.	morning
amp	ampule
amt	amount
aq	water
A.U.	both ears
b.i.d.; bid; BID	twice a day
BSA	body surface area
$\overline{c}$	with
cap; caps	capsule; capsules
cc	cubic centimeter
d	day
dil	dilute
disc; D.C.	discontinue
dr; ʒ	dram
D5W; D_5W	dextrose 5% in water
D/RL	dextrose $\overline{c}$ Ringer's lactate solution
D.W.	distilled water

elix	elixir
fl; fld	fluid
Gm; g; gm; G	gram
gr	grain
gtt; gtts	drop; drops
h; hr	hour
H.S.; h.s.; hs	at bedtime; hour of sleep
I.D.; ID	intradermal
I.M.; IM	intramuscular
I.V.; IV	intravenous
IVP; IV push	intravenous push or bolus
IVPB	intravenous piggyback
Kg; kg	kilogram
K.O.; KVO; TKO	keep open, keep vein open, to keep open
L; ℓ	liter
lb	pound
M; m	meter
mEq; meq	milliequivalent
mg	milligram
mL	milliliter
mm	millimeter
m; $\mathfrak{m}$; min	minim
m^2; M^2	square meter
μg; mcg	microgram
N & V	nausea and vomiting
NaCl	sodium chloride
noc; noct; n	night
NPO	nothing by mouth
N.S.; NS; N/S	normal saline (NaCl 0.9%)
½ NS	half strength normal saline (sodium chloride 0.45%)
O.D.	right eye
o.d.; q.d.; qd	every day
oh, o.h.	every hour
O.S.	left eye
OTC	over the counter
O.U.	both eyes
oz; ℥	ounce
p.c.; pc	after meals
per	by means of
Per os; p.o.; po	by mouth, orally
P.M.; p.m.	afternoon
PRN; p.r.n.	whenever necessary
pt; O	pint
q̄; q	every

q.d.	every day
q.o.d.; qod	every other day
q.h.; qh	every hour
q.2.h.; q2h	every 2 hours
q.3.h.; q3h	every 3 hours
q.4.h.; q4h	every 4 hours
q.6.h.; q6h	every 6 hours
q.8.h.; q8h	every 8 hours
q.12.h.; q12h	every 12 hours
q.i.d., qid, QID	four times a day
qt	quart
R; ®	rectal
R.L.; R/L	Ringer's lactate
Rx	take
$\bar{s}$	without
s.c.; subc; subq; sc	subcutaneous
S.L.; subl	sublingual
s.o.s.	once if necessary
sol	solution
sp	spirit
ss; $\overline{ss}$	one half
S & S	swish and swallow
stat; STAT	immediately
supp	suppository
syr	syrup
tab; tabs	tablet; tablets
tbsp; T; tbs	tablespoon
t.i.d.; tid; TID	three times a day
tinct; tr	tincture
tsp; t	teaspoon
U; u	unit
ung	ointment
vag	vaginal

Interpretation of Medication Orders

The medication order should contain:

a. The name of the medication.

b. The amount *or* dosage of the medication.

c. The route of administration and/or how the medication is to be given.

d. When the medication is to be administered.

e. Special or additional instructions for the person preparing the medication (this is not always essential for the order to be complete).

Using your knowledge of the symbols and abbreviations on the previous page, work through the following examples.

Example 1

Seconal Sodium® gr iss p.o. q.d. at h.s. repeat s.o.s.

  a. What is the name of the medication?
  Seconal Sodium (secobarbital sodium)

  b. What is the dosage to be administered?
  One and one half grains (gr iss)

  c. How is the medication to be administered?
  By mouth or orally (p.o.)

  d. When is the medication to be administered?
  Every day (q.d.) at bedtime (h.s.)

  e. What other directions are given to the preparer?
  Can repeat the drug one time if necessary (s.o.s.)

Example 2

1000 cc D_5W q.8.h. IV add 20 mEq Potassium Chloride to every third bottle.

  a. What are the names of the medications?
  Dextrose five percent (5%) in water (D_5W) and Potassium Chloride

  b. What is the dosage of each medication?
  1000 cubic centimeters (cc) of the D_5W and 20 milliequivalents (mEq) of the Potassium Chloride

  c. How are the medications to be administered?
  Intravenous (IV)

  d. When are the medications to be administered?
  Every 8 hours (q.8.h.)

  e. What other directions are given to the preparer?
  The Potassium Chloride will be mixed with every third bag or bottle of D_5W

☐ Practice Problems

Test your understanding of abbreviations and symbols by interpreting the following medication orders:

1. Torecan® (thiethylperazine maleate) 10 mg IM q.8.h. PRN for N&V.
    a. What is the name of the medication?

    b. What is the dosage of the medication?

    c. How is the medication to be administered?

    d. When is the medication to be administered?

    e. What other directions are given to the preparer?

2. Sodium Sulamyd® (sulfacetamide sodium) 30% gtts ii O.S. b.i.d.
    a. What is the name of the medication?

    b. What is the amount of the medication?

    c. How is the medication to be administered?

    d. When is the medication to be administered?

3. Foscavir® (foscarnet sodium) 60 mg per kg of body weight IVPB infuse over 1 hr q8h.

   a. What is the name of the medication?

   b. What is the dosage of the medication?

   c. How is the medication to be administered?

   d. What is the rate of administration of the medication?

   e. When is the medication to be administered?

4. Aspirin® (aspirin) supp gr x stat and q.4.h. p.r.n. for temperature over 101°F orally.

   a. What is the name of the medication?

   b. What is the dosage of the medication?

   c. How is the medication to be administered?

   d. When is the medication to be administered?

  e. What other directions are given to the preparer?

5. Minocin® (minocycline hydrochloride) syr 0.04 Gm po q.i.d. disc after 5 days.

  a. What is the name of the medication?

  b. What is the dosage of the medication?

  c. How is the medication to be administered?

  d. When is the medication to be administered?

  e. What other directions are given to the preparer?

6. NPH® (isophane insulin suspension) U-100 insulin 40 U subc q.d. in a.m.

  a. What is the name of the medication?

  b. What is the dosage of the medication?

  c. How is the medication to be administered?

    d. When is the medication to be administered?

7. Stat IV of 250 mL of 0.9% NaCl c̄ 2 mg of Isuprel (isoproterenol) to infuse at 3 mcg/minute.

    a. What are the names of the medications?

    b. What are the amounts of each medication?

    c. How are the medications to be administered?

    d. What is the rate of administration of the medications?

    e. When are the medications to be administered?

8. Inderal® (propranolol hydrochloride) 10 mg p.o. t.i.d. a.c. and at h.s.

    a. What is the name of the medication?

    b. What is the amount of the medication?

    c. How is the medication to be administered?

   d. When is the medication to be administered?

9. Cyanocobalamin injection 1000 μg IM q̄ month.
   a. What is the name of the medication?

   b. What is the dosage of the medication?

   c. How is the medication to be administered?

   d. When is the medication to be administered?

10. Follow present IV c̄ 1000 cc 0.45 NS c̄ i amp Berocca-C® IV at 125 mL/hr then D.C. I.V.
    a. What are the names of the medications?

    b. What are the amounts of the medications?

    c. How are the medications to be administered?

    d. When are the medications to be administered?

e. What other directions are given to be the preparer?

□ **Answers**

1. a. Torecan
    b. Ten milligrams
    c. Intramuscular
    d. Every 8 hours whenever necessary
    e. To be given for nausea and vomiting
2. a. Sodium Sulamyd 30%
    b. Two drops
    c. By drop in left eye
    d. Twice a day
3. a. Foscavir
    b. Sixty milligrams per each kilogram of body weight
    c. By intravenous piggyback
    d. Infuse over 1 hour (*Note:* This information may not be in the physician's order. The literature may need to be read to obtain the rate of infusion of the IV drug.)
    e. Every 8 hours
4. a. Aspirin
    b. Ten grains
    c. Suppository
    d. Immediately and every 4 hours whenever necessary
    e. To be given only if the oral temperature is above 101°F
5. a. Minocin syrup
    b. Four one hundredths of a gram
    c. By mouth
    d. Four times a day
    e. The drug is to be discontinued after 5 days or 20 doses
6. a. N.P.H. U 100 insulin
    b. Forty units
    c. Subcutaneously
    d. Every day in the morning
7. a. 0.9% sodium chloride and Isuprel
    b. 250 milliliters of the 0.9% NaCl and 2 milligrams of the Isuprel
    c. Intravenous
    d. Three micrograms of the Isuprel over each minute
    e. Immediately

8. a. Inderal
   b. Ten milligrams
   c. By mouth
   d. Three times a day before meals and at bedtime
9. a. Cyanocobalamin injection
   b. One thousand micrograms
   c. Intramuscular
   d. One time every month
10. a. One half normal saline solution and Berocca-C
    b. 1000 cubic centimeters of the ½NS and one ampule of Berocca-C
    c. Intravenous
    d. After completion of the present intravenous
    e. The fluid is to be infused at a rate of 125 milliliters per hour and intravenous fluids are to be discontinued after completion of this solution

Interpretation of Medication Labels

To prepare, administer, and store medications safely, information on medication labels must be carefully read and interpreted. The kind of information found on the label will vary, but basic information such as the drug name(s), strength, form, expiration date, and lot number will be present on the label (Fig. 4.1). The circular accompanying the drug, references, or the pharmacist must be consulted if additional information is needed.

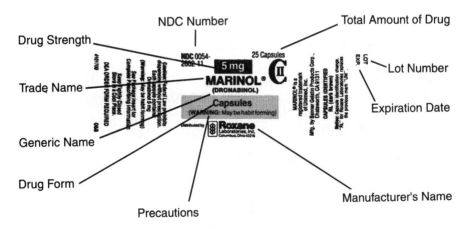

Figure 4.1.

Trade Name

This is the name given by the pharmaceutical company that manufactured the drug. It is also referred to as the brand name or proprietary name. The trade name is printed in capital letters or the first letter is capitalized. The symbol ® that follows the name signifies that it is the property of the manufacturer. The same medication may be produced by several companies, each using its own trade name.

Generic Name

This the chemical name of the drug. It is the officially accepted name as listed in the National Formulary. A drug may have several trade names, but only one generic name. The generic name may be the only name on the label when the drug is prepared and dispensed in its generic form.

Drug Strength

This identifies the dosage of the drug in the form dispensed in the container. Liquid forms are expressed in strength (eg, mEq, Gm, mcg) of the drug contained in a specific volume (eg, 3 mL, tsp i, 500 mL). Solid forms are expressed in strength (eg, gr, mg, g) of the drug contained in one tablet, one capsule, one transdermal patch, a tube of ointment, or other form of drug. Manufacturers produce a variety of different strengths of a drug per solid and/or liquid form. It is important that this information on the label be read carefully. For example, Corgard® is manufactured in strengths of 20, 40, 80, 120, and 160 mg per tablet.

Drug Form

This describes the type of preparation (eg, tablet, solution, injectable, lyophilized, transdermal system, ointment) of the drug as prepared by the manufacturer. A specific drug may be manufactured in a variety of forms.

Administration Route

The label may identify how the medication is to be administered (eg, oral, sublingual, IV, subcutaneous). The label may identify the route with a generic term such as injectable or "for injection." The literature or circular accompanying the drug would need to be read to determine the safe parenteral route(s). The oral route may not be specified if the drug comes in capsule or tablet form.

Total Amount of Drug

This defines the total amount of drug in solid (eg, 100 tablets, 24 packages) or liquid (eg, 2 mL, 1000 mL) form in the container. The number may also indicate the total volume of the drug that will be available after the drug has been reconstituted.

Expiration Date

Refers to the date after which the drug is no longer effective. The drug should not be administered after this date.

Lot Number

Identifies the batch of drugs from which this medication came when it was manufactured. This number provides specific product identification if problems should occur with the drug.

National Drug Code (NDC) Number

A number used by the manufacturer to identify the drug and the method of packaging.

Manufacturer's Name

Name of the pharmaceutical company that produced this drug.

Other information that may be found on labels includes the usual dosage, how to store the drug, and the type and amount of solution if the drug needs to be reconstituted or further diluted. Precautions related to the administration, preparation, or storage may also be added to the label (eg, dilute before use; single dose vial for IM use only; protect from light; may be habit forming). The literature or circular should always be read to obtain information that is not on the label but is needed to safely prepare and administer the drug.

☐ **Practice Problems**

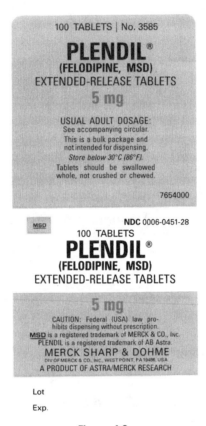

Figure 4.2.

1. Use Figure 4.2 to answer the following:

   a. Trade name _____

   b. Generic name _____

   c. Drug strength _____

   d. Drug form _____

   e. Total amount of drug _____

   f. NDC number _____

g. Expiration date _____

h. Lot number _____

i. Manufacturer _____

j. Precautions _____

_____

_____

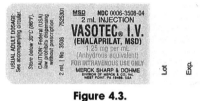

Figure 4.3.

2. Use Figure 4.3 to answer the following:

a. Trade name _____

b. Generic name _____

c. Drug strength _____

d. Total amount of drug _____

e. Drug form _____

f. Administration route _____

g. Manufacturer _____

h. Precautions _____

_____

_____

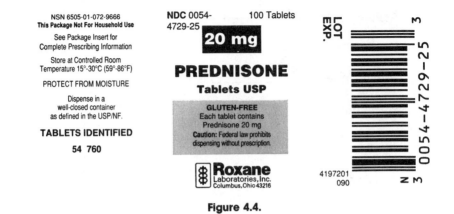

Figure 4.4.

3. Use Figure 4.4 to answer the following:

   a. Trade name _____

   b. Generic name _____

   c. Drug strength _____

   d. Drug form _____

   e. Administration route _____

   f. Total amount of drug _____

   g. Manufacturer _____

   h. Expiration date _____

   i. Lot number _____

   j. Precautions _____

   _____

   _____

   _____

   _____

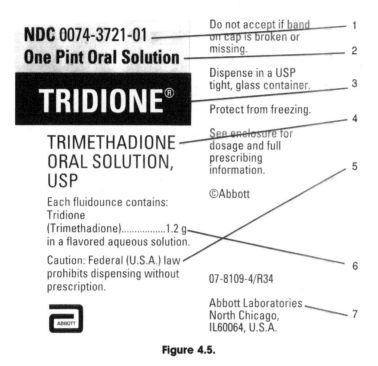

Figure 4.5.

4. Use Figure 4.5 to answer the following:

   a. Identify the kinds of information printed on the label.

   b. Each fluid ounce contains what strength of the drug Tridione?

   c. What is the total volume of Tridione in this container?

   d. What kind of solution is the drug prepared in?

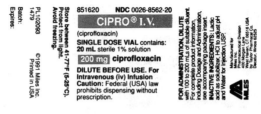

Figure 4.6.

5. Use Figure 4.6 to answer the following:

   a. Trade name _____

   b. Generic name _____

   c. Drug strength _____

   d. Drug form _____

   e. Total amount of drug _____

   f. Administration route _____

   g. What kind of container is the drug dispensed in? _____

   h. What directions are given for preparation of the medication for ad-

      ministration? _____

   i. What information is provided regarding storage of this drug?

      _____

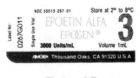

Figure 4.7.

6. Use Figure 4.7 to answer the following:

   a. Trade name _____

b. Generic name _____

c. Drug strength _____

d. Drug form _____

e. Administration route _____

f. Total volume of drug _____

g. Kind of container the drug is dispensed in _____

NDC 0002-7265-01
VIAL No. 7265

ADD-Vantage® Vial
KEFZOL®
STERILE CEFAZOLIN
SODIUM, USP

Equiv. to

Cefazolin

ACTIVATE AND MIX
KEFZOL® STERILE CEFAZOLIN **500 mg**
SODIUM, USP

For Intravenous Use
Each ADD-Vantage Vial contains: 500 mg of Cefazolin
and 0.04% Polysorbate 80.
The total sodium content is
approximately 24 mg (1.05
mEq sodium ion) per 500 mg
of KEFZOL.
Usual Adult Dose: 250 mg
to 1 g every six to eight
hours.—See literature.
For I.V. solution—See literature for directions.

Prior to **Reconstitution:**
Protect from Light.
Store at 15° to 30°C (59°
to 86°F).
After Reconstitution: If kept
at room temperature, use
within 24 hours.
Package/Patent Pending
(vials and diluent
containers, Abbott Laboratories).
ADD-Vantage®
WV-4663 AMX
Eli Lilly & Co., Indpls, IN 46285, U.S.A.
Exp. Date/Control No.

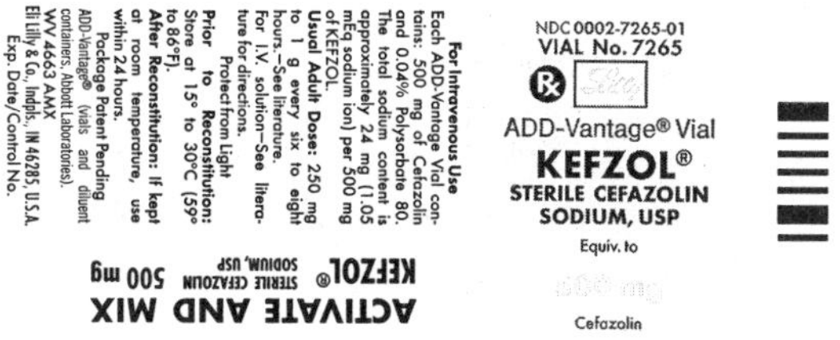

Figure 4.8.

7. Use Figure 4.8 to answer the following:

a. Trade name _____

b. Generic name _____

c. Drug strength _____

d. Administration route _____

e. Kind of container the drug is dispensed in _____

f. Manufacturer _____

g. Procedure for reconstitution of the drug _____

☐ **Answers**

1. a. Plendil®
   b. Felodipine, MSD
   c. 5 mg per tablet
   d. Extended-release tablet
   e. 100 tablets
   f. 0006-0451-28
   g. This is a sample label; the expiration date is not listed in the space provided
   h. This is a sample label; the lot number is not printed in the space provided
   i. Merck Sharp, & Dohme
   j. Directs reader to the accompanying circular to obtain the usual adult dosage. Store below 30°C or 86°F. Tablets should not be crushed or chewed, but swallowed whole. Federal law prohibits dispensing without a prescription.

2. a. Vasotec® IV
   b. Enalaprilat, MSD
   c. 1.25 mg per mL
   d. 2 mL in container (*Note:* Because this container holds 2 mL of this drug, the total strength of the drug in this container is 2.5 mg. An error could be made if the total volume was withdrawn when the strength ordered was 1.25 mg.)
   e. Liquid injectable
   f. Intravenous (IV)
   g. Merck Sharp & Dohme
   h. Usual adult dose: see accompanying circular. Store below 30°C (86°F). Federal law prohibits dispensing without prescription. For intravenous use only.

3. a. No trade name, drug prepared in generic form
   b. Prednisone
   c. 20 mg per tablet
   d. Tablet
   e. Administration route is not stated on the label. This drug is given by the oral route.
   f. 100 tablets
   g. Roxane Laboratories
   h. Not listed—this is a sample label
   i. Not listed—this is a sample label
   j. Federal law prohibits dispensing without prescription. Store at controlled room temperature 15–30°C (59–86°F). Protect from moisture.

4. a. 1). Administration route
      2). Drug form
      3). Trade name
      4). Generic name
      5). Precautions
      6). Drug strength per volume
      7). Manufacturer
   b. 1.2 gram of Tridione per ounce
   c. One pint
   d. Flavored aqueous solution
5. a. Cipro® IV
   b. Ciprofloxacin
   c. 200 mg per 20 mL
   d. Liquid solution
   e. 20 mL
   f. Intravenous (IV) infusion
   g. Single-dose vial
   h. Dilute with 100 to 200 mL of suitable diluent. Directs preparer to read accompanying package insert for additional information to prepare and administer this drug.
   i. Store between 41 and 77°F. Protect from light. Avoid freezing.
6. a. Epogen®
   b. Epoetin alfa
   c. 3000 units per milliliter
   d. Liquid solution
   e. Not printed on label—obtain from the literature
   f. 1 milliliter
   g. Single-use vial
7. a. Kefzol®
   b. Cefazolin sodium
   c. 500 mg
   d. Intravenous
   e. Add-Vantage vial
   f. Lilly
   g. Not printed on the label—obtain from the literature

Use of the Proportion Formula to Calculate Equivalent Units of Measure

The metric, apothecaries', and household systems are used interchangeably in clinical situations. Proportions can be used when one must convert from one unit of measure to another within the same system (eg, tsp to tbsp) or to convert from one system to another (eg, gr to mg).

Need for Conversion

The need for conversion occurs in various situations.

1. The strength of the drug ordered by the physician and the drug available for administration are not in the same unit of measure.

Example

Order: Codeine gr ½.
Drug Available: Codeine 30 mg per tablet.

Example

Order: Ampicillin 0.5 Gm.
Drug Available: Ampicillin 500 mg per capsule.

Before one can determine the quantity of the drug to be given, the prescribed dosage or the dosage available must be converted to its equivalent unit.

2. A more accurate measure of the quantity of the dosage to administer is desired.

Example

Drug available in mL.
Desire measurement in ℞ (minims).

3. The strength of the drug may be ordered according to the weight of the

patient in kilograms or the weight of the patient in kilograms is needed to determine a safe dosage.

Example

Order: Aminophylline 6 mg/kg of body weight.
Patient's weight: 108 pounds.

Before one can determine the dosage to be given, the patient's weight in pounds must be converted to kilograms.

Known equivalent ratios are used in setting up the proportion. An *equivalent* is a unit of measure that is considered to be of equal or approximately equal value to a unit of measure expressed in the same system or in a different system of measure.

$$15 \text{ grains } = \quad 1 \text{ gram}$$
$$16 \text{ minims } = \quad 1 \text{ milliliter}$$
$$1 \text{ ounce } = 30 \text{ milliliters}$$

TABLE 5.1. Summary of Essential Equivalents

Household	Apothecary	Metric
	Volume	
1 tsp = 5 mL	1 fl dr = 4 mL[a]	5 mL = 1 tsp
3 tsp = 1 tbsp	4 drams = ½ ounce	15 mL = 1 tbsp
1 tbsp = ½ oz or	8 drams = 2 tbsp (1 oz)	30 mL = 2 tbsp
15 mL	16 minims = 1 mL	1 mL = 16 minims[c]
2 tbsp = 1 oz or	1 pint[b] = 16 oz or	500 mL = 0.5 liter or
30 mL	480 mL	1 pint
Teacup = 6 oz	1 quart[b] = 32 oz or	1000 mL = 1 liter or
Glass or cup = 8 oz	960 mL	1 quart

Weight

$$\tfrac{1}{60} \text{ grain } = 1 \text{ mg}$$
$$1 \text{ grain } = 60 \text{ mg or } 0.060 \text{ Gm}$$
$$15 \text{ grains } = 1 \text{ gram or } 1000 \text{ mg}$$
$$2.2 \text{ lbs } = 1 \text{ kg}$$
$$1 \text{ mg } = 1000 \text{ μg}$$

[a] The fluid dram is equivalent to 4 rather than 5 mL. The use of 5 mL as an equivalent measurement was for the convenience of calculations. Equipment used for measuring liquids show a difference in a dram and a teaspoon. Always check the dosage and volume carefully and clarify the order with the physician.
[b] The pint is considered to be 500 cc and the quart is considered to be 1000 cc when used in medication orders.
[c] Sixteen (16) minims is used as the equivalent rather than 15 since the equipment for dispensing medications is calibrated in 16 minims per mL.

The units of measure in one system are not exactly equal in value to the units in another system. For example, 1 grain may equal from 0.06 grams to 0.065 grams or 60 milligrams to 65 milligrams. If the nurse is not consistent in using equivalents, the answer to problems could vary enough to make significant differences in the desired amount of the drug. *It is important to remember that conversions from one system to another are only approximate equivalents.* The equivalents identified in Table 5.1 are the accepted standards used in converting from one system of measure to another. Only the most commonly used equivalents are included and should be memorized.

Setting Up a Proportion

Remember the following points when setting up a proportion:

1. A ratio describes a relationship that exists between two numbers. The ratio 16:1 may describe any one of the following relationships:

   Sixteen ounces is the same as (or equal to) *one* pint.

   There are *sixteen* ounces in *one* pound.

   Sixteen milligrams of the drug are contained in *one* tablet.

2. A proportion consists of two ratios which have the same value. The proportion defines the relationship that exists between the two ratios. When the numbers in each ratio are properly labeled, for example:

   $$16 \text{ oz} : 1 \text{ pt} :: 32 \text{ oz} : 2 \text{ pts}$$

   This proportion would describe the following relationship:

   Sixteen ounces equals one pint; therefore thirty-two ounces would equal two pints.

3. Each ratio in a proportion must exhibit the *same* relationship. *The second ratio of the proportion must follow in the same sequence* to maintain the same relationship as the first ratio. Label each term of each ratio to prevent error.

   Correct sequence/relationships:
   16 oz : 1 pt :: 32 oz : 2 pts
   Sequence of first ratio is oz to pt.
   Sequence of second ratio is also oz to pt.

   Incorrect sequence/relationships:
   16 oz : 1 pt :: 2 *pts* : 32 *oz*
   16 oz : 1 pt :: 32 *tsp* : 1 *qt*

In the following examples note how each of the ratios is expressed and the sequence of the relationships in each proportion.

Example 1

If it requires three teaspoons (3 tsp) to fill one tablespoon (1 tbsp), then nine teaspoons (9 tsp) are required to fill three tablespoons (3 tbsp).

3 tsp : 1 tbsp : : 9 tsp : 3 tbsp

Example 2

One cup contains eight ounces; therefore twenty-four ounces equal three cups.

1 cup : 8 oz : : 3 cups : 24 oz

Example 3

One kilogram (1 kg) equals two and two-tenths pounds (2.2 lbs); therefore five kilograms (5 kg) equal eleven pounds (11 lbs).

1 kg : 2.2 lbs : : 5 kg : 11 lbs

Setting Up a Proportion to Convert Within and Between Systems

When converting from one unit of measure to another, set up each ratio of the proportion using the following steps:

1. The first ratio of the proportion contains the known equivalent.

Known Unit of Measure : Known Equivalent Unit of Measure

1000 mg : 1 Gm

2. The second ratio of the proportion contains the desired unit of measure and the unknown equivalent. The "unknown" equivalent is represented by the symbol "X." The ratio containing the unknown equivalent can be placed in either the first or second ratio, but it is preferable to state the known relationship in the first ratio and the unknown relationship in the second ratio.

Desired Unit of Measure : Unknown Equivalent

500 mg : X Gm

The terms of the second ratio are stated in the same sequence/position (mg to Gm) as the first ratio (mg to Gm), and therefore maintain the same relationship as expressed in the first ratio.

3. When the two ratios are set in proportion, the equation appears as follows:

		Known		Desired		
Known Unit	:	Equivalent	::	Unit of	:	Unknown
of Measure		Unit of Measure		Measure		Equivalent

$$1000 \text{ mg} \quad : \quad 1 \text{ Gm} \quad :: \quad 500 \text{ mg} \quad : \quad X \text{ Gm}$$

The proportion is now properly stated and ready to be solved.

$$1000 \text{ mg} : 1 \text{ Gm} :: 500 \text{ mg} : X \text{ Gm}$$

$$1000 \text{ X} = 500$$

$$X = 0.5 \text{ Gm}$$

Note

Label your answer to remind you what unit of measure your answer represents.

Proof:

$$1000 \text{ mg} : 1 \text{ Gm} :: 500 \text{ mg} : 0.5 \text{ Gm}$$

$$500 = 500$$

Examples of Conversions Using the Proportion

Example 1

How many ounces are there in one and one-half pints?

a. Express in proportion.

Known Unit	Known Equivalent		Desired Unit	Unknown
of Measure	Unit of Measure	::	of Measure	Equivalent

$$1 \text{ pt} : 16 \text{ oz} :: 1.5 \text{ pt} : X \text{ oz}$$

b. Solve to obtain unknown equivalent.

$$1 \text{ pt} : 16 \text{ oz} :: 1.5 \text{ pt} : X \text{ oz}$$

$$1 \text{ X} = 24$$

$$X = 24 \text{ oz}$$

c. Proof:

$$1 \text{ pt} : 16 \text{ oz} :: 1.5 \text{ pt} : 24 \text{ oz} \qquad 24 \text{ oz} = 24 \text{ oz}$$

Example 2

Five-tenths of a milliliter (0.5 mL) is the equivalent of how many minims?

a. Express in proportion.

Known Unit . Known Equivalent .. Desired Unit . Unknown
of Measure : Unit of Measure :: of Measure : Equivalent

1 mL : 16 ℳ :: 0.5 mL : X ℳ

b. Solve to obtain unknown equivalent.

1 mL : 16 ℳ :: 0.5 mL : X ℳ

1 X = 8

X = 8 ℳ (ℳ viii)

c. Proof:

1 mL : 16 ℳ :: 0.5 mL : 8 ℳ   8 ℳ = 8 ℳ

Example 3

Twenty milligrams (20 mg) is equal to what fraction of a grain?

a. Express in proportion.

60 mg : 1 gr :: 20 mg : X gr

b. Solve to obtain unknown equivalent.

60 mg : 1 gr :: 20 mg : X gr

60 X = 20

$$X = \frac{20}{60} = \frac{1}{3} \text{ grain}$$

In the apothecaries' system, parts of whole numbers, other than one half, are expressed as common fractions. When it is evident that the answer will be less than one, compute the problem using common fractions.

c. Proof:

60 mg : 1 gr :: 20 mg : ⅓ grain   20 mg = 20 mg

☐ **Practice Problems**

Directions
Use the proportion formula to convert each item to the appropriate equivalent.

1. ¼ gr   = _____ mg   2. 120 mg   = _____ Gm

3. 0.05 Gm = _____ gr   4. 55 lbs   = _____ kg

5. 250 µg = _____ mg   6. 0.3 mL   = _____ ℳ

7. 4 dr   = _____ mL   8. 45 mL   = _____ oz

9. 1½ oz = _____ dr   10. 1.25 L   = _____ mL

11. 20 mL = _____ tsp   12. 1½ gr   = _____ g

13. 0.2 mg = _____ gr   14. 2500 mg = _____ Gm

15. 30 kg = _____ lbs   16. 24 ℳ   = _____ cc

17. 12 oz = _____ cc   18. 0.003 mg = _____ µg

19. 4 tsp = _____ dr   20. 1000 mL = _____ pts

21. 165 lbs = _____ kg   22. 1.5 tsp   = _____ cc

23. 3 gr   = _____ mg   24. 1⅓ oz   = _____ tsp

25. 0.006 g = _____ mg   26. 32 mL   = _____ ꝫ

27. 15 µg = _____ mg   28. 3 cups   = _____ mL

29. 7½ gr = _____ Gm   30. 1.5 qts   = _____ oz

☐ **Answers**

1. 1 gr : 60 mg :: gr ¼ : X mg

     X = 15 mg

   (if equivalent 15 gr : 1000 mg was used, X = 16.6 mg)

2. 1000 mg : 1 Gm : : 120 mg : X Gm

$$1000\ X\ =\ 120$$

$$X\ =\ 0.120\ Gm$$

3. 1 Gm : 15 gr : : 0.05 Gm : X gr

$$X\ =\ 0.75\ gr\ or\ gr\ \tfrac{3}{4}$$

(if equivalent 1 gr : 0.060 or gr $\frac{1}{60}$: 0.001 Gm, X = gr $\frac{5}{6}$)

4. 2.2 lbs : 1 kg : : 55 lbs : X kg

$$2.2\ X\ =\ 55$$

$$X\ =\ 25\ kg$$

5. 1000 μg : 1 mg : : 250 μg : X mg

$$1000\ X\ =\ 250$$

$$X\ =\ 0.25\ mg$$

6. 1 mL : 16 ♏ : : 0.3 mL : X ♏

$$1\ X\ =\ 4.8\ or\ 5\ ♏$$

(Because of the size of a minim, you would round this off to the nearest whole minim.)

7. 1 dr : 4 ml : : 4 dr : X mL

$$X\ =\ 16\ mL$$

8. 30 ml : 1 oz : : 45 mL : X oz

$$30\ X\ =\ 45$$

$$X\ =\ 1\tfrac{1}{2}\ or\ ℥\ iss$$

9. ½ oz : 4 dr : : 1½ oz : X dr

$$\tfrac{1}{2}\ X\ =\ 6$$

$$X\ =\ 12\ dr\ or\ ℨ\ xii$$

10. 1 L : 1000 mL : : 1.25 L : X mL

$$X\ =\ 1250\ mL$$

11. 5 ml : 1 tsp : : 20 mL : X tsp

$$5\ X\ =\ 20$$

$$X\ =\ 4\ tsp$$

12. $15 \text{ gr} : 1 \text{ g} :: 1\frac{1}{2} \text{ gr} : X \text{ g}$

$$15 \text{ X} = 1\frac{1}{2} (1.5)$$

$$X = 0.1 \text{ g}$$

(if equivalent 1 gr : 0.06 g, X = 0.09 g)

13. $60 \text{ mg} : 1 \text{ gr} :: 0.2 \text{ mg} : X \text{ gr}$

$$60 \text{ X} = 0.2$$

$$X = 0.2 \div 60$$

$$X = \frac{2}{10} \times \frac{1}{60} = \frac{2}{600} = \frac{1}{300} \text{ gr}$$

14. $1000 \text{ mg} : 1 \text{ Gm} :: 2500 \text{ mg} : X \text{ Gm}$

$$1000 \text{ X} = 2500$$

$$X = 2.5 \text{ Gm}$$

15. $1 \text{ kg} : 2.2 \text{ lbs} :: 30 \text{ kg} : X \text{ lbs}$

$$1 \text{ X} = 66 \text{ lbs}$$

16. $16 \text{ m} : 1 \text{ cc} :: 24 \text{ m} : X \text{ cc}$

$$16 \text{ X} = 24$$

$$X = 1.5 \text{ cc}$$

17. $1 \text{ oz} : 30 \text{ cc} :: 12 \text{ oz} : X \text{ cc}$

$$1 \text{ X} = 360 \text{ cc}$$

18. $1 \text{ mg} : 1000 \text{ μg} :: 0.003 \text{ mg} : X \text{ μg}$

$$1 \text{ X} = 3 \text{ μg}$$

19. $1 \text{ tsp} : 1 \text{ dr} :: 4 \text{ tsp} : X \text{ dr}$

$$1 \text{ X} = 4 \text{ drams or ʒ iv}$$

20. $500 \text{ mL} : 1 \text{ pt} :: 1000 \text{ mL} : X \text{ pt}$

$$500 \text{ X} = 1000$$

$$X = 2 \text{ pt}$$

21. $2.2 \text{ lbs} : 1 \text{ kg} :: 165 \text{ lbs} : X \text{ kg}$

$$2.2 \text{ X} = 165$$

$$X = 75 \text{ kg}$$

22. 1 tsp : 5 cc :: 1.5 tsp : X cc

$$1 X = 7.5 \text{ cc}$$

23. 1 gr : 60 mg :: 3 gr : X mg

$$1 X = 180 \text{ mg}$$

(if equivalent 15 gr : 1000 mg, X = 200 mg)

24. ½ oz : 3 tsp :: 1⅓ oz : X tsp

$$\tfrac{1}{2} X = 4$$

$$X = 8 \text{ tsp}$$

(remember to invert the fraction, ½ becomes ⅖₁, then multiply by the 4)

25. 1 g : 1000 mg :: 0.006 g : X mg

$$1 X = 6 \text{ mg}$$

26. 4 mL : 1 dr :: 32 mL : X dr

$$4 X = 32$$

$$X = 8 \text{ dr or } \mathfrak{z} \text{ viii}$$

27. 1000 μg : 1 mg :: 15 μg : X mg

$$1000 X = 15$$

$$X = 0.015 \text{ mg}$$

28. 1 cup : 8 oz :: 3 cup : X oz

$$1 X = 24 \text{ oz}$$

1 oz : 30 mL :: 24 oz : X mL

$$1 X = 720 \text{ mL}$$

29. 15 gr : 1 Gm :: 7½ gr : X Gm

$$15 X = 7\tfrac{1}{2} \ (7.5)$$

$$X = 0.5 \text{ Gm}$$

(if equivalent 1 gr : 0.06 Gm, X = 0.45 Gm)

30. 1 qt : 32 oz :: 1.5 qt : X oz

$$1 X = 48 \text{ oz}$$

If you missed more than 5 problems, review the chapter before proceeding to the next practice problems.

☐ **Additional Practice**

Directions

Express each problem in a proportion and solve to obtain the desired equivalent.

1. One-sixth grain (gr ⅙) is the equivalent of how many milligrams?

2. If there are one one-thousandths gram (0.001 Gm) in one milligram (1 mg), how many grams are there in two-hundred milligrams (200 mg)?

3. How many minims will you administer to equal seven-tenths milliliter (0.7 mL) of a drug?

4. One one-hundredths milligram (0.01 mg) is the equivalent of how many micrograms?

5. The physician orders five grains (gr v) of a drug that is available in grams. How many grams equal the dosage ordered?

6. If one tablet contains three hundred and twenty milligrams (320 mg) of a drug, how many grams would this be equal to?

7. How many milliliters are there in two drams (ʒ ii)?

8. A dropper is calibrated to disperse twenty drops (gtts xx) per milliliter (1 mL). Fifteen drops (gtts xv) from this calibrated dropper would be the equivalent of what portion of a milliliter?

9. A child weighs fifty-four pounds (54 lbs). What is this child's weight in kilograms?

10. The patient drank twenty-one ounces (℥ xxi) of water. How many cubic centimeters of water did this patient drink?

11. A bottle contains eight ounces (℥ viii) of liquid medication. This is equivalent to how many drams?

12. A patient received three liters (3 L) of intravenous fluid over 24 hours. How many cubic centimeters of fluid did this patient receive for the 24 hours?

13. The medication is available in one-hundred-and-fifty milligrams (150 mg) per one tablet. This is equivalent to how many grains?

14. How many pounds are there in ninety kilograms (90 kg)?

15. Seventy-five-one-hundredths gram (0.75 Gm) of a drug is to be administered to a patient. How many grains of this drug will the patient receive?

16. If eight ounces (℥ viii) equals one glass, then one glass equals how many cubic centimeters?

17. How many milligrams are equal to fifteen one-thousandths gram (0.015 g)?

18. One and twenty-five hundredths cubic centimeters (1.25 cc) is the equivalent of how many minims?

19. If the patient took six drams (ʒ vi) of a drug, how many milliliters of the drug did the patient take?

20. The label states that this five-milliliter bottle contains five-hundred milligrams (500 mg) of a drug. How many micrograms are there in this five-milliliter bottle?

21. The physician prescribed seventy-five-one-hundredths gram (0.75 Gm) of a drug to be given in three equally divided doses over a 24-hour period of time. The drug is available in milligrams. How many milligrams will the patient receive per each dose?

22. The patient reported he drank six ounces (℥ vi) of juice, eight ounces of coffee (℥ viii), and four ounces (℥ iv) of water. How many milliliters of fluid in total did this patient drink?

23. How many milligrams equal grains one-eighth (gr ⅛)?

24. A baby, who weighs eleven pounds (11 lbs), is to receive one-eighth grain (gr ⅛) of a drug per kilogram of body weight. How many kilograms does this baby weigh?

25. Four tablespoons of fluid equals how many ounces?

26. One grain (gr i) of a prescribed drug is contained in sixty-two-one-hundredths milliliter (0.62 mL). How many minims will you prepare to equal the prescribed dose?

27. Four-one-hundredths gram (0.04 Gm) is the equivalent of how many micrograms?

28. A patient is to have three fluid drams (℥ iii) of a drug. This is equivalent to how many teaspoons?

29. If there are four-tenths gram (0.4 Gm) in six grains (gr vi), how many grams are there in one-fifth grain (gr ⅕)?

30. If five milliliters (5 mL) equals one teaspoon, one-fourth teaspoon (¼ tsp) equals how many minims?

☐ **Answers**

1. gr $\frac{1}{60}$: 1 mg :: gr $\frac{1}{6}$: X mg

   $\frac{1}{60}$ X = $\frac{1}{6}$

   X = 10 mg

2. 1 mg : 0.001 Gm :: 200 mg : X Gm

   1 X = 0.2 Gm

3. 1 mL : 16 ♏ :: 0.7 mL : X ♏

   X = 11.2 or 11 ♏

4. 1 mg : 1000 µg :: 0.01 mg : X µg

   1 X = 10 µg

5. 15 gr : 1 Gm :: 5 gr : X Gm

   15 X = 5

   X = 0.33 Gm

   (if equivalent 1 gr : 0.06 Gm, then X = 0.30 Gm)

6. 1 Gm : 1000 mg :: X Gm : 320 mg

   1000 X = 320

   X = 0.32 Gm

7. 1 dram : 4 ml :: 2 dram : X mL

   1 X = 8 ml

8. 20 gtts : 1 ml :: 15 gtts : X mL

   20 X = 15

   X = 0.75 ml

9. 2.2 lbs : 1 kg :: 54 lbs : X kg

   2.2 X = 54

   X = 24.5 kg

10. 1 oz : 30 cc :: 21 oz : X cc

    1 X = 630 cc

11. 1 oz : 8 dr :: 8 oz : X dr

    1 X = 64 drams

12. 1 L : 1000 cc : : 3 L : X cc

$$1 X = 3000 \text{ cc}$$

13. 15 gr : 1000 mg : : X gr : 150 mg

$$1000 X = 2250$$

$$X = 2.25 \text{ gr (gr } 2\tfrac{1}{4})$$

(if equivalent 1 gr : 60 mg, then X = gr iiss)

14. 2.2 lbs : 1 kg : : X lbs : 90 kg

$$1 X = 198 \text{ lbs}$$

15. 1 gr : 0.06 Gm : : X gr : 0.75 Gm

$$0.06 X = 0.75$$

$$X = 12.5 \text{ gr or gr xiiss}$$

(if equivalent 1 Gm : 15 gr, then X = 11.25 gr)

16. 30 cc : 1 oz : : X cc : 8 oz

$$1 X = 240 \text{ cc (1 glass} = 240 \text{ cc)}$$

17. 1000 mg : 1 g : : X mg : 0.015 g

$$1 X = 15 \text{ mg}$$

18. 16 ℳ : 1 cc : : X ℳ : 1.25 cc

$$1 X = 20 \text{ ℳ (ℳ xx)}$$

19. 4 mL : 1 dram : : X mL : 6 drams

$$1 X = 24 \text{ mL}$$

20. 1 mg : 1000 µg : : 500 mg : X µg

$$1 X = 500,000 \text{ µg}$$

21. 3 doses : 0.75 Gm : : 1 dose : X Gm

$$3 X = 0.75$$

$$X = 0.25 \text{ Gm/dose}$$

1 Gm : 1000 mg : : 0.25 Gm : X mg

$$1 X = 250 \text{ mg}$$

22. 6 oz + 8 oz + 4 oz = 18 oz (℥ xviii) total fluid in ounces.

1 oz : 30 mL : : 18 oz : X mL

$$1 X = 540 \text{ mL}$$

23. $\frac{1}{60}$ gr : 1 mg : : $\frac{1}{8}$ gr : X mg

$\quad\quad$ $\frac{1}{60}$ X = $\frac{1}{8}$

$\quad\quad\quad$ X = 7.5 mg

(if equivalent 15 gr : 1000 mg, X = 8.3 mg)

24. 2.2 lbs : 1 kg : : 11 lbs : X kg

$\quad\quad$ 2.2 X = 11

$\quad\quad\quad$ X = 5 kg

25. 2 tbsp : 1 oz : : 4 tbsp : X oz

$\quad\quad$ 2 X = 4

$\quad\quad\quad$ X = 2 oz ($\natural$ ii)

26. 1 mL : 16 ♏ : : 0.62 mL : X ♏

$\quad\quad$ 1 X = 9.92 ♏ or ♏ x

27. 1 Gm : 1000 mg : : 0.04 Gm : X mg

$\quad\quad$ 1 X = 40 mg

1 mg : 1000 μg : : 40 mg : X μg

$\quad\quad$ 1 X = 40,000 μg

28. 1 dr : 1 tsp : : 3 dr : X tsp

$\quad\quad$ 1 X = 3 tsp

29. 0.4 Gm ($\frac{4}{10}$) : 6 gr : : X Gm : $\frac{1}{5}$ gr

$\quad\quad$ 6 X = $\frac{1}{5}$ × $\frac{4}{10}$ ($\frac{2}{25}$)

$\quad\quad\quad$ X = $\frac{2}{25}$ × $\frac{1}{6}$ = $\frac{2}{150}$ = 0.013 Gm

$\quad\quad\quad\quad$ OR

0.4 Gm : 6 gr : : X Gm : 0.2 gr

$\quad\quad$ 6 X = 0.08

$\quad\quad\quad$ X = 0.013 Gm

30. 1 mL : 16 ♏ : : 5 mL : X ♏

$\quad\quad$ 1 X = 80 ♏

1 tsp : 80 ♏ : : $\frac{1}{4}$ tsp : X ♏

$\quad\quad$ 1 X = 20 ♏ (♏ xx)

Calculation of Oral Medications

Forms of Oral Medication

Medications taken by mouth come in a variety of liquid and solid forms. Liquid forms include syrups, elixirs, and suspensions. Tablets and capsules are the usual solid forms. Drugs in powder form, which are dissolved prior to administration, are also available for oral administration.

Each of these forms contain a specific strength (weight unit of measure) of a drug (Fig. 6.1). Liquid forms are expressed in strength (eg, mg, gr, Gm, mEq, μg) of the drug contained in a specific volume (eg, 30 mL, ℥ i, tsp i). Calibrated medication cups (Fig. 6.2), droppers (Fig. 6.3), or syringes can

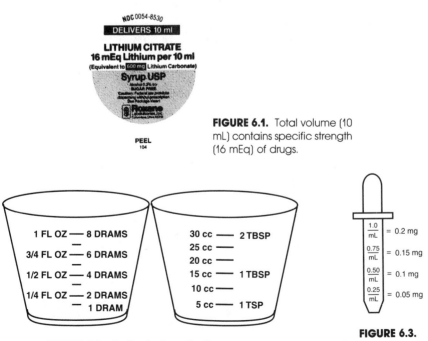

FIGURE 6.1. Total volume (10 mL) contains specific strength (16 mEq) of drugs.

FIGURE 6.2. Calibrated medication cups.

FIGURE 6.3. Calibrated dropper.

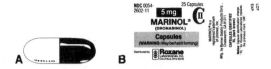

FIGURE 6.4. **A.** Capsule contains medication in powder, liquid, or oil form encased in a gelatin shell. **B.** Label denotes the total strength of the drug (5 mg) per capsule. If the ordered amount is less than the available dose (5 mg), there is no way to safely open the capsule and accurately measure the contents of the capsule; therefore, the order should be clarified.

be used to measure liquid medications. The medication cup is usually calibrated in mL, cc, tsp, tbsp, dr, and oz. The medication cup is not calibrated to measure less than 1 dram or to measure volumes that fall between the calibrations on the container. To measure volumes below 1 dram or for a more accurate measure, a hypodermic syringe without the needle or a manufactured oral syringe can be used. Droppers that accompany the medication may be calibrated in milliliters or in dosages that represent the strengths usually ordered.

Solid forms are expressed in strength (eg, mg, gr, Gm, µg) of the drug contained in one tablet or capsule (Fig. 6.4).

Tablets that are scored in halves or quarters may be divided to give a portion of the total strength of the drug (Fig. 6.5).

The medication order specifies the dosage or strength of the drug to be administered to the patient. The order may not identify the *number* of tablets or *amount* of solution of the medication to be administered to equal the strength ordered.

> Order: Artane® 2 mg p.o. tid with meals.
> Order: Artane elixir 3 mg p.o. tid with meals.

The nurse must compare the ORDER with the AVAILABLE medication to determine the quantity (number of tablets or volume) of the drug to administer. Often the amount to give is easily identified.

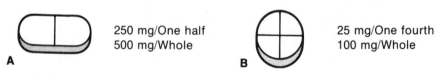

A   250 mg/One half
     500 mg/Whole

B   25 mg/One fourth
     100 mg/Whole

FIGURE 6.5. **A.** Each one half of the tablet contains one half (250 mg) of the total strength (500 mg) of the drug. **B.** Each one fourth of the tablet contains one fourth (25 mg) of the total strength (100 mg) of the drug.

Order: Artane (trihexyphenidyl HCl) 2 mg p.o. tid with meals.
Available: Artane 2 mg per scored tablet.

The strength of the drug ordered is the same as the dosage available. One tablet would be administered three times a day with meals.

At other times, the quantity to give is not easily identified. The nurse would need to use calculations to determine the amount of the available drug that would equal the ordered dosage.

Order: Artane 2.5 mg p.o. tid with meals.
Available: Artane 5 mg per scored tablet.

The amount available per tablet exceeds the ordered amount.

Order: Artane elixir 3 mg p.o. tid with meals.
Available: Artane elixir 2 mg per 5 mL.

The amount available per measured volume is less than the ordered amount.

The drug may also be available in various strengths per tablet or volume of solution. For example, Artane is available in 2 mg and 5 mg per scored tablet. The nurse would have to determine which strength or combinations of strengths to use based on the dosage ordered before calculating the quantity to administer.

With certain oral drugs, the medication order will specify the number of tablets or amount of solution of the medication to be administered and NOT the strength of the drug.

Gelusil® tab i p.o. q4h PRN.
Milk of magnesia 30 mL p.o. h.s.

The drugs prescribed in these types of orders are usually available in only one strength, or the medication contains a combination of drugs of various strengths. It is important to be familiar with these medications in order to know when to question a medication order that does not specify the strength of the drug.

To safely and accurately calculate the correct dosage, the proportion formula is recommended and will be used throughout this text whenever possible for the following reasons:

1. All problems, with the exception of some intravenous medication calculations and pediatric problems, can be solved by this method.

2. Writing the problem as a proportion clarifies what is known and available and what information is unknown and desired.

3. The problem can be proved by substituting the answer for the unknown.

4. The nurse does not have to remember a variety of formulas or whether to divide or multiply certain numbers.

5. The proportion can be used to convert the prescribed dosage or the dosage available to its equivalent unit of measure.

When the physician prescribes an oral medication, the proportion formula can be used to determine:

• How many or what portion of a tablet of the available drug to administer to the patient to equal the dosage prescribed by the physician.

• How many ounces, drams, milliliters, teaspoons, or drops of the available liquid medication to administer to the patient to equal the dosage prescribed by the physician.

Proportion Formula

$$\begin{array}{ccc} \text{Dosage} & \text{Known No. of} & \text{Dosage} & \text{Unknown No. of} \\ \text{Available} & \text{Tablets/Capsules} & \text{Prescribed} & \text{Tablets/Capsules} \end{array}$$

$$5 \text{ mg} \quad : \quad 1 \text{ tab} \quad :: \quad 2.5 \text{ mg} \quad : \quad X \text{ tab}$$

OR

$$\begin{array}{ccc} \text{Dosage} & \text{Known Volume} & \text{Dosage} & \text{Unknown Volume} \\ \text{Available} & \text{(mL, tsp, oz)} & \text{Prescribed} & \text{(mL, tsp, oz)} \end{array}$$

$$2 \text{ mg} \quad : \quad 5 \text{ mL} \quad :: \quad 3 \text{ mg} \quad : \quad X \text{ mL}$$

Example 1

Order: Cylert® (pemoline) 37.5 mg q a.m. p.o.
Available: Cylert labeled as in Figure 6.6.

How many Cylert 18.75-mg tablets should you administer to equal the dosage prescribed (37.5 mg)?

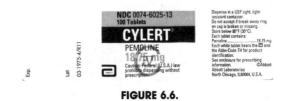

FIGURE 6.6.

$$\frac{Dosage}{Available} : \frac{Known\ No.}{of\ Tablets} :: \frac{Dosage}{Prescribed} : \frac{Unknown\ No.}{of\ Tablets}$$

$$18.75\ mg : 1\ tab :: 37.5\ mg : X\ tab$$

$$18.75\ X = 37.5$$

$$X = 2\ tab$$

The nurse should administer 2 tablets of Cylert (18.75 mg/tab).

Example 2

Order: Cardizem® SR (dilfiazem hydrochloride) gr 1½ p.o. bid.
Available: Cardizem SR 90 mg per capsule.

The prescribed dosage is in a unit of measure that is different from the unit of measure of the available drug. The nurse must convert the prescribed dosage to the same unit of measure as that of the available drug, or convert the available drug dosage to the same unit of measure as that of the prescribed dosage.

How many grains are equal to 90 mg?

$$\frac{Known}{Equivalent} :: \frac{Unknown}{Equivalent}$$

$$60\ mg : 1\ gr :: 90\ mg : X\ gr$$

$$60\ X = 90$$

$$X = 1½\ gr$$

Cardizem 90 mg per capsule is the same as Cardizem gr 1½. The prescribed dosage and the available drug dosage are now in the same unit of measure.

How many capsules of Cardizem 90 mg per capsule will you administer to equal the prescribed dosage (90 mg)?

$$\frac{Dosage}{Available} : \frac{Known}{Volume} :: \frac{Dosage}{Prescribed} : \frac{Unknown}{Volume}$$

$$90\ mg : 1\ cap :: 90\ mg : X\ cap$$

$$90\ X = 90$$

$$X = 1\ cap$$

The nurse should administer one Cardizem 90-mg capsule.

Example 3

Order: Amoxil® (amoxicillin) 125 mg p.o. q.8.h.
Available: Amoxil 250 mg per tsp.

How many or what portion of a tsp of Amoxil (250 mg/tsp) will you administer to equal the prescribed dosage (125 mg)?

$$250 \text{ mg} : 1 \text{ tsp} :: 125 \text{ mg} : X \text{ tsp}$$

$$250 X = 125$$

$$X = 0.5 \text{ tsp}$$

To obtain a more accurate measure of the amount of solution to administer to equal the dosage prescribed, convert the 0.5 tsp to milliliters.

$$1 \text{ tsp} : 5 \text{ mL} :: 0.5 \text{ tsp} : X \text{ mL}$$

$$1 X = 2.5 \text{ mL}$$

The nurse should administer 2.5 mL of Amoxil (250 mg/tsp) to equal the prescribed dosage (125 mg).

This conversion could have been done prior to calculating the volume of drug to be given by substituting the equivalent 5 mL for 1 tsp in the original problem.

$$250 \text{ mg} : 5 \text{ mL} :: 125 \text{ mg} : X \text{ mL}$$

$$250 X = 625$$

$$X = 2.5 \text{ mL}$$

It is advisable to use the equivalent 1 tsp : 5 mL when the available drug is measured in the metric system (250 mg).

☐ Practice Problems

Directions
Use the proportion formula to calculate the correct amount of drug to administer to the patient.

1. Order: NegGram Caplet® (nalidixic acid) 0.5 g p.o. qid.
   Available: NegGram 1 Gm per scored tablet.

   How many or what portion of a NegGram (1 Gm/tab) should you administer?

2. Order: Naprosyn® (naproxen) Suspension 375 mg p.o. b.i.d.
   Available: Naprosyn suspension 125 mg per 5 mL.

   a. How many milliliters of Naprosyn (125 mg/5 mL) should you administer?

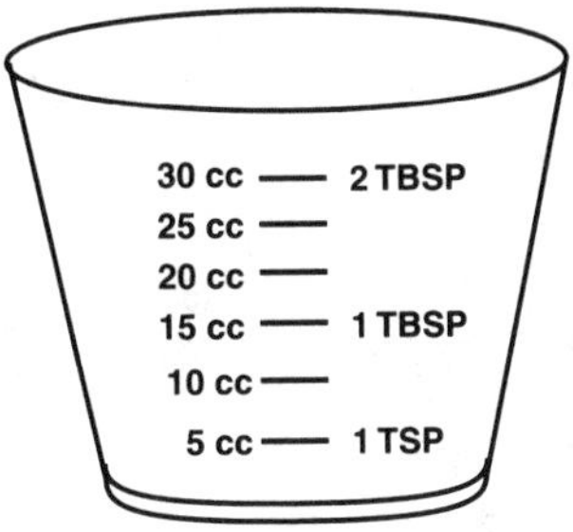

FIGURE 6.7.

b. On the medication cup in Figure 6.7, locate the volume you should administer to the patient.

3. Order: Phenobarbital® (phenobarbital) gr ¾ p.o. q.12.h.
Available: Phenobarbital gr iss per scored tablet.

How many or what portion of a tablet of the Phenobarbital (gr iss/ tab) should you administer?

4. Order: Calciferol® (ergocalciferol) 22,000 units p.o. q.d. 8 a.m.
Available: Calciferol oral solution 8000 units per 1 mL.

a. How many mL of Calciferol (8000 U/mL) equals the prescribed dose?

b. Your hospital is on military time. What is the time you would administer the drug?

5. Order: Rocaltrol® (calcitriol) 0.5 μg p.o. q.d. in a.m.
Available: Rocaltrol 0.25 μg per capsule.

How many capsules of Rocaltrol (0.25 mcg/cap) should you administer?

6. Order: DHT™ (dihydrotachysterol) 250 mcg po daily.
   Available: Two containers of DHT tablets labeled as shown in Figure 6.8.

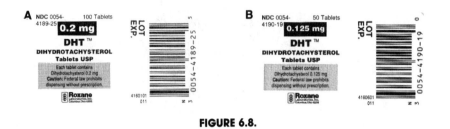

FIGURE 6.8.

a. How many mg equal 250 mcg?

b. What strength tablet should you use to prepare the prescribed dosage?

(Place the answer from b in the space provided in c.)

c. How many or what portion of a tablet of DHT (_____ mg/tab) should you administer?

7. Order: Tegopen® (cloxacillin sodium) oral solution 375 mg po q6h.
   Available: Tegopen oral solution 125 mg/5 mL.

a. How many tbsp equals 5 mL?

b. How many tbsp of Tegopen (125 mg/_____ tbsp) should the patient take?

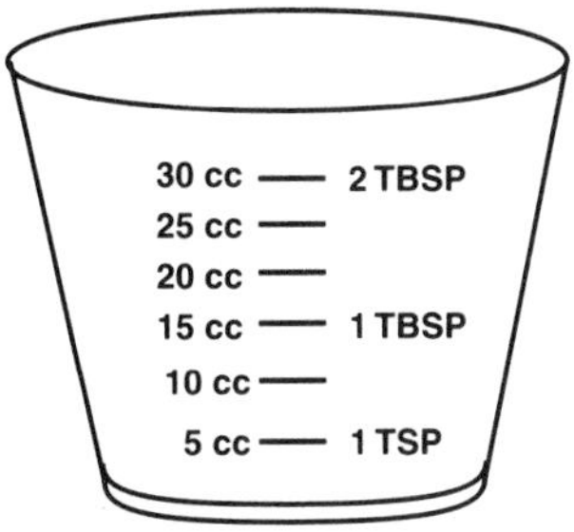

FIGURE 6.9.

   c. On the medication container in Figure 6.9, locate the volume in tbsp that you would administer to equal the dosage ordered.

8. Order: Armour Thyroid® (thyroid) gr ½ p.o. daily.
   Available: Armour Thyroid gr ¼ per tablet, gr 1 per tablet, and gr 2 per tablet.

   a. What strength tablet will you use to prepare the prescribed dose?

   b. How many tablets of Armour Thyroid (_____ gr/tab) should you administer?

9. Order: Biaxin® (clarithromycin) 0.5 g p.o. q12h.
   Available: Biaxin 250 mg per tablet.

   How many or what portion of Biaxin 250 mg per tablet will the patient receive?

10. Order: Ultracef® (cefradoxil) suspension 0.750 Gm p.o. b.i.d.
    Available: Ultracef suspension 125 mg/5 mL.

    a. How many Gm equals 125 mg?

b. How many mL of Ultracef suspension (_____ Gm/5 mL) should you administer?

c. How many oz of Ultracef suspension equals the prescribed dose?

11. Order: Synthroid® (levothyroxine sodium) 37.5 μg p.o. q.d. in a.m.
    Available: A bottle of Synthroid scored tablets labeled as shown in Figure 6.10.

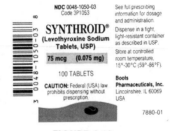

FIGURE 6.10.

How many or what portion of a tablet of Synthroid (_____ μg/tab) should you administer?

12. Order: Pravachol® (pravastatin sodium) gr ⅓ p.o. q h.s.
    Available: Pravachol 10 mg per tablet.

    a. How many grains are there in 10 mg?

    b. How many tablets of Pravachol (gr _____/tab) should you administer?

13. Order: Mebaral® (mephobarbital) 0.2 g p.o. q.d.
    Available: Mebaral gr ¾ per tablet.

    a. How many g are equal to gr ¾?

    b. How many tablets of Mebaral (_____ g/tab) should you administer?

14. Order: Benadryl® elixir (diphenhydramine hydrochloride) 37.5 mg
    q.12.h. p.o.
    Available: Benadryl elixir 12.5 mg per 5 mL.

    a. How many milliliters of Benadryl (12.5 mg/5 mL) should you administer?

    b. How many or what portion of an ounce of Benadryl (12.5 mg/5 mL) should you administer to equal the prescribed dosage?

15. Order: Tridione® (trimethadione oral suspension) 300 mg p.o. t.i.d.
    Available: Tridione labeled as shown in Figure 6.11A.

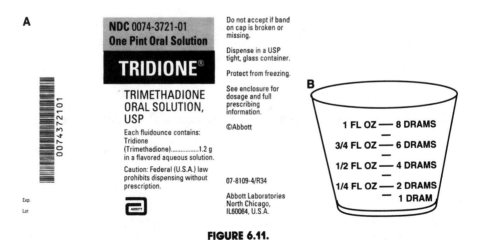

FIGURE 6.11.

Draw a line on the medication container (Fig. 6.11B) to identify the volume you would pour to equal the dosage of Tridione ordered.

16. Order: SSKI® (potassium iodide oral solution) 300 mg p.o. q.i.d. in one glass of water.
    Available: SSKI oral solution 1 Gm/mL.

    a. How many ℞ of SSKI (_____ mg/_____ ℞) should you administer to equal the prescribed dose?

    b. How many doses per day will the patient receive?

17. Order: Pyrazinamide 0.75 g p.o. q6h.
    Available: Pyrazinamide 500 mg scored tablets.
    Usual dosage is 20–35 mg/kg/day in three or four equally divided doses.

    Patient's weight: 176 lbs.

    a. How many tablets should you administer?

    b. Is this patient receiving a usual dosage of Pyrazinamide per day?

18. Order: Marinol® (dronabinol) 7500 mcg p.o. q4h PRN for N&V.
    Available: Two containers of Marinol labeled as shown in Figure 6.12.

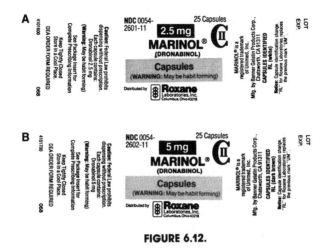

FIGURE 6.12.

Which capsules and how many of each will you prepare to equal the dosage ordered?

19. Order: Furoxone® (furazolidone) suspension 0.1 Gm p.o. q.i.d.
    Available: Bottle containing 473 mL of Furoxone. Each tbsp equals
         50 mg.

    a. How many mL of Furoxone should you administer to equal the
       prescribed dose?

    b. How many Gm of Furoxone will be available in this bottle at the
       end of the third day of therapy?

20. Order: Roxanol 100™ (morphine sulfate oral solution) gr ⅔ q4h p.r.n.
         pain.
    Available: Roxanol 100™ labeled as shown in Figure 6.13 and accom-
         panied with the calibrated spoon.

a. Draw a line on the calibrated spoon (Fig. 6.13) to identify how many mg of Roxanol 100 you will prepare to equal the dosage ordered.

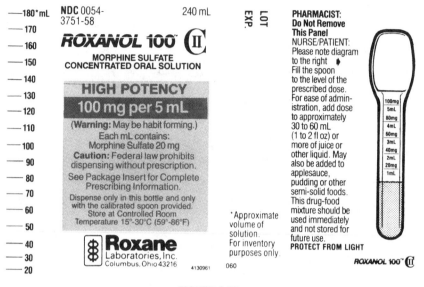

FIGURE 6.13.

b. How many mL will the patient receive?

21. Order: Lodine® (etodolac) 400 mg p.o. q6h prn pain.
    Available: Lodine 200 mg per capsule.

    a. How many capsules will the patient receive to equal the desired dose?

    b. The patient received the last dose at 1700. At what hour can the patient again receive the Lodine?

    c. The total daily dose should not exceed 20 mg per kg of body weight. This patient weighs 132 lbs. How many mg of Lodine can this patient safely receive in one day?

22. Order: Lithium Citrate syrup 8 mEq p.o. b.i.d.
    Available: A unit dose of Lithium Citrate labeled as shown in Figure
       6.14.

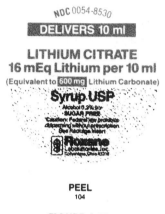

FIGURE 6.14.

Draw a line on the medication container shown in Figure 6.15 to identify the volume you would pour to equal the dosage of Lithium Citrate
ordered.

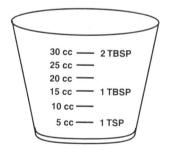

FIGURE 6.15.

23. Order: Lanoxin® (digoxin) tablets 0.375 mg p.o. STAT.
    Available: Lanoxin 125 μg, 250 μg, and 500 μg per scored tablet.

   a. Which Lanoxin tablet will you use to prepare the prescribed dose?

b. How many tablets of Lanoxin (_____ µg/tab) should the patient receive?

24. Order: Choledyl® (oxtriphylline) elixir 3.1 mg/kg p.o. q.6.h.
    Available: Choledyl elixir 100 mg/5 mL.
    Patient's weight: 121 lbs.

    How many mL of Choledyl should the patient receive?

25. Order: DHT™ (dihydrotachysterol intensol) 0.15 mg daily.
    Available: Bottle of DHT solution with calibrated dropper. Figure 6.16 shows the bottle label.

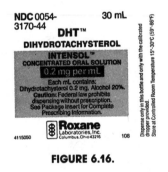

FIGURE 6.16.

a. How many mg of DHT are contained in this bottle?

b. How many mL of DHT will the patient receive to equal the prescribed dose?

c. On the dropper in Figure 6.17, locate the amount you should administer to the patient.

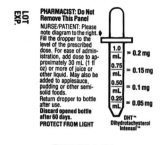

FIGURE 6.17.

26. Order: Vascor® (bepridil HCL) 0.4 Gm p.o. q.d.
    Available: Vascor 200 mg per scored tablet, 300 mg per tablet, and 400 mg per tablet.

    Select the correct tablet(s) to equal the dosage ordered.

27. Order: Ethmozine® (moricizine HCL) 0.9 g p.o. over 24 hr period in 3 equally divided doses.
    Available: Ethmozine 300 mg per tablet.

    a. How many g of Ethmozine should you administer for each dose?

    b. How many tablets of Ethmozine (300 mg) should you administer for each dose?

    c. At what frequency should you administer each dose?

    d. If the first dose was given at 0800, identify in military time when the patient will receive the second and third dose.

28. Order: Depakene® Syrup (valproic acid) 400 mg p.o. q.12.h.
    Available: Depakene Syrup 250 mg per 5 mL. The literature accompanying this drug states that the daily dosage of Depakene should not exceed 15 mg per kg of body weight.
    Patient's weight: 88 lbs.

    a. How many kg does this patient weigh?

    b. Using the dosage (15 mg/kg/body wt) defined in the literature, what is the maximum daily dose of Depakene that this patient could receive?

    c. Is the prescribed dosage below or above the dosage defined in the literature?

29. Order: Ilosone® suspension (erythromycin estolate) 0.75 Gm p.o. q.i.d.
    Available: Sixteen ounces of Ilosone suspension. Each 5 mL contains 250 mg.

    a. How many Gm are equal to 250 mg?

    b. How many mL of Ilosone suspension (_____ Gm/5 mL) should you administer?

    c. How many mL are equal to ℥ xvi?

    d. How many doses of Ilosone are contained in this bottle?

30. Order: Septra Suspension® (trimethoprim and sulfamethoxazole) 1 oz
p.o. q.6.h.
Available: Septra Suspension. Each 5 mL contains 40 mg of trimethoprim and 200 mg of sulfamethoxazole.

a. How many mg of trimethoprim and sulfamethoxazole is the patient
receiving per day?

b. Is the prescribed dosage above or below the recommended dosage?
The product information recommended dosage for a patient with
this disease is 20 mg/kg trimethoprim and 100 mg/kg of sulfamethoxazole per 24 hr in 4 equally divided doses. This patient
weighs 60 kg.

☐ **Answers**

1. 1 Gm : 1 tab :: 0.5 Gm : X tab

$$1 X = 0.5$$

$$X = \frac{1}{2} \text{ tablet}$$

2. a. 125 mg : 5 mL :: 375 mg : X mL

$$125 X = 1875$$

$$X = 15 \text{ mL}$$

b.

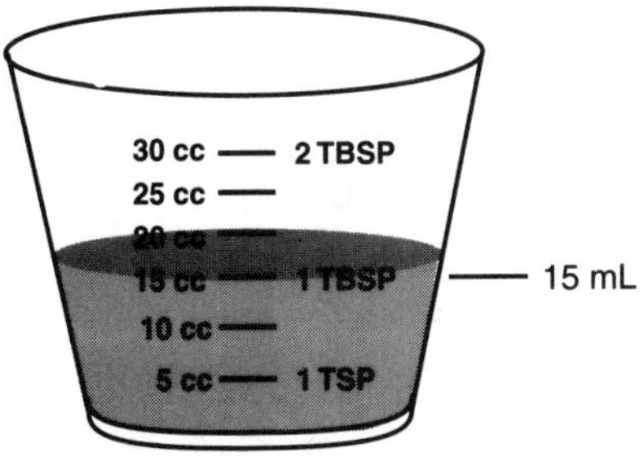

FIGURE 6.18.

3. 1½ gr : 1 tab :: ¾ gr : X tab

$$1\frac{1}{2} X = \frac{3}{4}$$

$$X = \frac{3}{4} \times \frac{2}{3} = \frac{2}{4} \text{ or } \frac{1}{2} \text{ tab}$$

4. a. 8000 U : 1 mL :: 22,000 U : X mL

$$8000 \ X = 22,000$$

$$X = 2.75 \text{ or } 2.8 \text{ mL}$$

b. 0800 hour

Note

If your answer is a whole number and a decimal, the general rule is to first carry the answer out 2 decimal places and if the second place is 5 or greater, increase the number to the left by 1 (18.75 = 18.8). Second, look to see if the answer is related to tablets or liquids. If the answer was 1.8 tablets you would have to give 2 tablets, because it is impossible to accurately divide the tablet into .8. On the other hand, if the answer was 1.8 cc, you would administer 1.8 cc—this can easily be measured in a syringe. Remember that if the drug is available in a form that can be divided into fractional doses, you would only round the answer to the nearest $\frac{1}{10}$, and if the drug is *not* available in a form easily divided, you would administer a dosage as close as possible to the prescribed dose (1.2 tablet = 1 tablet or 2.7 tabs = 3 tabs).

5. 0.25 mcg : 1 cap :: 0.5 mcg : X cap

$$0.25 \ X = 0.5$$

$$X = 2 \text{ caps}$$

6. a. 1000 mcg : 1 mg :: 250 mcg : X mg

$$1000 \ X = 250$$

$$X = 0.25 \text{ mg}$$

b. 0.125 mg/tablet

c. 0.125 mg : 1 tab :: 0.25 mg : X tab

$$0.125 \ X = 0.25$$

$$X = 2 \text{ tabs}$$

7. a. 15 mL : 1 tbsp :: 5 mL : X tbsp

$$15 \ X = 5$$

$$X = \frac{1}{3} \text{ tbsp}$$

b. 125 mg : $\frac{1}{3}$ tbsp :: 375 mg : X tbsp

$$125 \ X = {}^{375}\!/_{3}$$

$$X = 1 \text{ tbsp}$$

c.

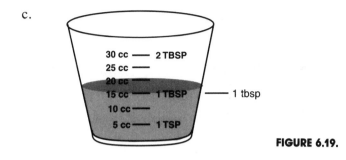

FIGURE 6.19.

8. a. Armour Thyroid gr ¼/tab

b. ¼ gr : 1 tab :: ½ gr : X tab

$$\frac{1}{4} X = \frac{1}{2}$$

X = 2 tablets

Note

Tablets are not scored so the 1 gr tablet could not be broken in half.

9. 1 g : 1000 mg :: 0.5 g : X mg

1 X = 500 mg

250 mg : 1 tab :: 500 mg : X tab

250 X = 500

X = 2 tabs

10. a. 1000 mg : 1 Gm :: 125 mg : X Gm

1000 X = 125

X = 0.125 Gm

b. 0.125 Gm : 5 ml :: 0.750 Gm : X mL

0.125 X = 3.75

X = 30 mL

c. 30 mL = 1 oz = prescribed dose

11. 75 μg : 1 tab :: 37.5 μg : X tab

75 X = 37.5

X = 0.5 tab

12. a. 60 mg : 1 gr :: 10 mg : X gr

$$60 X = 10$$

$$X = \frac{1}{6} \text{ gr}$$

b. $\frac{1}{6}$ gr : 1 tab :: $\frac{1}{3}$ gr : X tab

$$\frac{1}{6} X = \frac{1}{3}$$

$$X = \frac{1}{3} \times \frac{6}{1}$$

$$X = 2 \text{ tabs}$$

13. a. 15 gr : 1 g :: $\frac{3}{4}$ gr : X g

$$15 X = \frac{3}{4}$$

$$X = \frac{1}{20} \text{ or } 0.05 \text{ g}$$

b. 0.05 g : 1 tab :: 0.2 g : X tab

$$0.05 X = 0.2$$

$$X = 4 \text{ tabs}$$

14. a. 12.5 mg : 5 mL :: 37.5 mg : X mL

$$12.5 X = 187.5$$

$$X = 15 \text{ mL}$$

b. 15 mL = $\frac{1}{2}$ oz or ℥ ss

or

12.5 mg : $\frac{1}{6}$ oz :: 37.5 mg : X oz

$$12.5 X = 6.25$$

$$X = 0.5 \text{ oz or } ℥ \text{ ss}$$

15. 1200 mg : 1 oz :: 300 mg : X oz

$$1200 X = 300$$

$$X = 0.25 \text{ oz } (\frac{1}{4} \text{ oz})$$

OR

1200 mg : 8 drams :: 300 mg : X drams

$$1200 X = 2400$$

$$X = 2 \text{ drams}$$

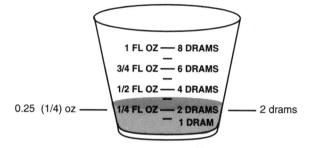

FIGURE 6.20.

16. a. 1000 mg (1 Gm) : 16 ℳ (1 mL) : : 300 mg : X ℳ

$$1000 \, X = 4800$$

$$X = 4.8 \text{ or } 5 \text{ ℳ}$$

b. 4 doses

17. a. 1 g : 1000 mg : : 0.75 g : X mg

$$1 \, X = 750 \text{ mg}$$

500 mg : 1 tab : : 750 mg : X tab

$$500 \, X = 750$$

$$X = 1.5 \text{ tabs}$$

b. 2.2 lbs : 1 kg : : 176 lbs : X kg

$$2.2 \, X = 176$$

$$X = 80 \text{ kg}$$

20 mg : 1 kg : : X mg : 80 kg

$$1 \, X = 1600 \text{ mg} = \text{lowest dosage}$$

35 mg : 1 kg : : X mg : 80 kg

$$1 \, X = 2800 \text{ mg} = \text{highest dosage}$$

750 mg : 1 dose : : X mg : 4 doses

$$1 \, X = 3000 \text{ mg}$$

Patient is receiving 200 mg more per day than the highest usual dose.

18. 1000 mcg : 1 mg : : 7500 mcg : X mg

$$1000 \, X = 7500$$

$$X = 7.5 \text{ mg}$$

Prepare one 5-mg capsule and one 2.5-mg capsule of Marinol to equal the dosage ordered.

19. a. 1000 mg : 1 Gm : : 50 mg : X Gm

$$1000 \ X = 50$$

$$X = 0.05 \ Gm$$

0.05 Gm : 1 tbsp : : 0.1 Gm : X tbsp

$$0.05 \ X = 0.1$$

$$X = 2 \ tbsp$$

1 tbsp : 15 mL : : 2 tbsp : X mL

$$1 \ X = 30 \ mL$$

b. 0.4 Gm : 1 day : : X Gm : 3 days

$$1 \ X = 1.2 \ Gm$$

0.05 Gm : 15 mL : : X Gm : 473 mL

$$15 \ X = 23.65$$

$$X = 1.58 \ Gm/bottle$$

1.58 Gm available
$$\underline{- \ 1.20 \ Gm \ administered}$$
0.38 Gm remaining

20. a. 1 gr : 60 mg : : ⅔ gr : X mg

$$1 \ X = {}^{120}\!/_{3} = 40 \ mg$$

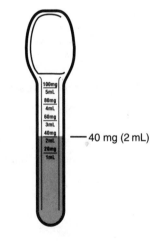

—40 mg (2 mL)

FIGURE 6.21.

b. 100 mg : 5 mL :: 40 mg : X mL

$$100 \text{ X} = 200$$

$$\text{X} = 2 \text{ mL}$$

21. a. 200 mg : 1 cap :: 400 mg : X cap

$$200 \text{ X} = 400$$

$$\text{X} = 2 \text{ capsules}$$

b. 2300 hours or 11 P.M.

c. 2.2 lbs : 1 kg :: 132 lbs : X kg

$$2.2 \text{ X} = 132$$

$$\text{X} = 60 \text{ kg}$$

20 mg : 1 kg :: X mg : 60 kg

$$1 \text{ X} = 1200 \text{ mg (total amount patient can}$$
$$\text{receive in a 24-hour period)}$$

22. 16 mEq : 10 mL :: 8 mEq : X mL

$$16 \text{ X} = 80$$

$$\text{X} = 5 \text{ mL (5 cc)}$$

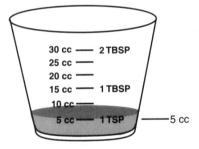

FIGURE 6.22.

23. a. 1 mg : 1000 μg :: 0.375 mg : X μg

$$1 \text{ X} = 375 \text{ μg}$$

250 μg scored tablet

b. 250 μg : 1 tab :: 375 μg : X tab

$$250 \text{ X} = 375$$

$$\text{X} = 1.5 \text{ tab}$$

Note

You always give the fewest tablets or least volume possible.

24. a. 2.2 lbs : 1 kg :: 121 lbs : X kg

    2.2 X = 121

    X = 55 kg

    3.1 mg : 1 kg :: X mg : 55 kg

    1 X = 170.5 mg

    100 mg : 5 mL :: 170.5 mg : X mL

    100 X = 852.5

    X = 8.52 or 8.5 mL

25. a. 0.2 mg : 1 mL :: X mg : 30 mL

    1 X = 6 mg

    b. 0.2 mg : 1 mL :: 0.15 mg : X mL

    0.2 X = 0.15

    X = 0.75 mL

    c.

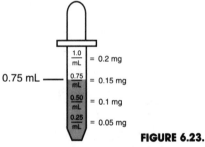

FIGURE 6.23.

26. 1 Gm : 1000 mg :: 0.4 Gm : X mg

    1 X = 400 mg

Administer one 400-mg tablet of Vascor. This selection prevents the patient from receiving 2 tablets to equal the dosage ordered.

27. a. 3 doses : 0.9 g :: 1 dose : X g

    3 X = 0.9

    X = 0.3 g

b. 1000 mg : 1 g :: 300 mg : X g

   $\qquad$ 1000 X = 300

   $\qquad$ X = 0.3 g

   $\qquad$ 0.3 g : 1 tab :: 0.3 g : X tab

   $\qquad$ X = 1 tab

c. 3 doses : 24 hr :: 1 dose : X hr

   $\qquad$ 3 X = 24

   $\qquad$ X = 8 hr or q.8.h.

d. The second dose would be administered at 1600 and the third dose at 2400.

28. a. 2.2 lbs : 1 kg :: 88 lbs : X kg

   $\qquad$ 2.2 X = 88

   $\qquad$ X = 40 kg

   b. 1 kg : 15 mg :: 40 kg : X mg

   $\qquad$ 1 X = 600 mg

   c. Prescribed dose (800 mg/day) is above the dosage defined in the literature (600 mg).

29. a. 1000 mg : 1 Gm :: 250 mg : X Gm

   $\qquad$ 1000 X = 250

   $\qquad$ X = 0.250 Gm

   b. 0.250 Gm : 5 mL :: 0.75 Gm : X mL

   $\qquad$ 0.250 X = 3.75

   $\qquad$ X = 15 mL

   c. 1 oz : 30 mL :: 16 oz : X mL

   $\qquad$ 1 X = 480 mL

   d. 15 mL : 1 dose :: 480 mL : X dose

   $\qquad$ 15 X = 480

   $\qquad$ X = 32 doses

30. a. 5 mL : 40 mg :: 30 mL (1 oz) : X mg

$$5 X = 1200$$

$$X = 240 \text{ mg trimethoprim}$$

240 mg : 1 dose :: X mg : 4 doses

$$1 X = 960 \text{ mg trimethoprim/day}$$

5 mL : 200 mg :: 30 mL : X mg

$$5 X = 6000$$

$$X = 1200 \text{ mg sulfamethoxazole}$$

1200 mg × 4 doses = 4800 mg sulfamethoxazole/day

b. 20 mg : 1 kg :: X mg : 60 kg

$$1 X = 1200 \text{ mg trimethoprim/day}$$

100 mg : 1 kg :: X mg : 60 kg

$$1 X = 6000 \text{ mg sulfamethoxazole/day}$$

Receiving below recommended dose.

If you missed more than 5 problems, review the chapter and the problems before starting next chapter.

Parenteral Drugs in Solution

Many of the parenteral drugs given by injection either intramuscularly (IM), subcutaneously (subc), or intradermally are prepared in liquid form by the drug manufacturer. The solution is contained in single-dose ampules, single- or multiple-dose vials, prefilled disposable syringes, single-dose cartridge injector units with needle attached, and other similar containers (Fig. 7.1).

The label on the container identifies the strength (eg, 0.4 mg, 1 Gm) of the drug in a specific volume of solution (eg, 0.5 mL, 1 mL). Milligrams, grams, grains, units, and micrograms are the unit of weight measures. The

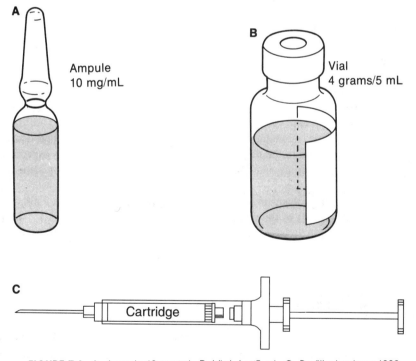

A. Ampule 10 mg/mL

B. Vial 4 grams/5 mL

C. Cartridge

FIGURE 7.1. A. Ampule 10 mg/mL. **B.** Vial 4 g/5 mL. **C.** Prefilled syringe 1000 U/mL.

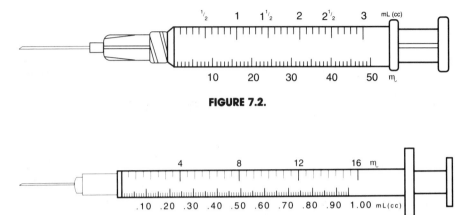

FIGURE 7.2.

FIGURE 7.3.

milliliter is the most common unit of volume measure used on the manufacturer's label. The label may define a specific dose per volume (eg, 10 mg/1 mL) or it may define the total strength of the drug in the container per total volume (eg, 20 mg/2 mL).

    Syringes (Fig. 7.2), used to measure parenteral drugs for administration, are calibrated in cubic centimeters (milliliters) and are available in a variety of sizes (eg, 1, 3, and 6 cc). The smaller syringes (eg, 2½ or 3 cc) are usually calibrated in tenths of a cubic centimeter (eg, 0.2, 0.3, 0.8 cc) and in minims. Single-dose cartridge units are usually calibrated in tenths of a cubic centimeter.

    The tuberculin (TB) syringe is a 1-milliliter syringe calibrated in tenths and hundredths of a milliliter (eg, 0.3 mL, 0.35 mL) and in minims (eg, 16.23 ℳ/1 mL). Such a syringe is shown in Figure 7.3.

    The tuberculin syringe can be used when the volume is less than 1 milliliter and a more precise measurement of the dosage is needed. The prescribed dosage volume can be calibrated to the nearest hundredth of a milliliter. This is especially important with certain drugs and when calculating dosages to be administered to infants and children.

    If the volume is greater than 1 milliliter, the dosage volume can be calibrated in minims or rounded off to the nearest tenth of a milliliter.

Using the Proportion Formula

When the physician prescribes a parenteral drug, the proportion formula can be used to determine what volume (eg, mL, cc, ℳ) of the available drug to administer to the patient to equal the prescribed dosage.

Example 1

Order: Demerol® (meperidine hydrochloride) 75 mg IM q.4.h. p.r.n. for pain.
Available: Demerol ampule labeled 100 mg per 2 mL.

How many mL of Demerol (100 mg/2 mL) should you administer to equal the prescribed dosage (75 mg)?

$$\frac{Dosage}{Available} : \frac{Known}{Volume} :: \frac{Dosage}{Prescribed} : \frac{Unknown}{Volume}$$

$$100 \text{ mg} : 2 \text{ mL} :: 75 \text{ mg} : X \text{ mL}$$

$$100 X = 150$$

$$X = 1.5 \text{ mL}$$

The nurse should administer 1.5 ml of Demerol (100 mg/2 mL).

Example 2

Order: Morphine sulfate (morphine sulfate) gr $\frac{1}{8}$ IM stat.
Available: Morphine sulfate ampule labeled 15 mg per 1 mL.

a. How many grains are equal to 15 mg?

$$Known \text{ Equivalent} :: Unknown \text{ Equivalent}$$

$$1 \text{ mg} : gr \tfrac{1}{60} :: 15 \text{ mg} : X \text{ gr}$$

$$1 X = \tfrac{15}{60}$$

$$X = \tfrac{1}{4} \text{ gr}$$

Morphine sulfate 15 mg/1 mL is the same as Morphine sulfate gr $\frac{1}{4}$/1 mL. The prescribed dosage and the available drug are now in the same unit of measure.

Note

When making conversions, convert the order to the available or the available to the order. Choose the one that is easiest for you.

b. How many mL of Morphine sulfate (gr $\frac{1}{4}$/mL) should you administer to equal the prescribed dosage (gr $\frac{1}{8}$)?

$$\frac{Dosage}{Available} : \frac{Known}{Volume} :: \frac{Prescribed}{Dosage} : \frac{Unknown}{Volume}$$

$$gr \tfrac{1}{4} : 1 \text{ mL} :: gr \tfrac{1}{8} : X \text{ mL}$$

$$\tfrac{1}{4} X = \tfrac{1}{8}$$

$$X = \tfrac{4}{8} \text{ or } 0.5 \text{ mL}$$

The nurse should administer 0.5 mL of Morphine sulfate gr $\frac{1}{4}$/mL.

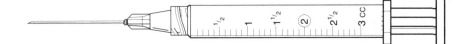

FIGURE 7.4.

c. Locate the amount of Morphine sulfate you should draw into the syringe in Figure 7.4 to equal the prescribed dosage.

Example 3

Order: Nebcin® (tobramycin sulfate) 3 mg per kg of body weight IM per day (24 hr) administered in 3 equal doses q.8.h.
Available: Nebcin, each vial containing 80 mg per 2 mL.
Patient's weight: 220 lbs.

a. How much does this patient weight in kg?

$$2.2 \text{ lbs} : 1 \text{ kg} :: 220 \text{ lbs} : X \text{ kg}$$

$$2.2 X = 220$$

$$X = 100 \text{ kg}$$

This patient weighs 100 kg.

b. What is the total dosage of Nebcin prescribed by the physician?

$$3 \text{ mg} : 1 \text{ kg} :: X \text{ mg} : 100 \text{ kg}$$

$$1 X = 300 \text{ mg}$$

Based on the patient's weight in kg, the physician has prescribed 300 mg of Nebcin to be given over a 24-hour period.

c. How many mg of Nebcin per each dose should the patient receive q.8.h.?

$$300 \text{ mg} : 3 \text{ doses} :: X \text{ mg} : 1 \text{ dose}$$

$$3 X = 300$$

$$X = 100 \text{ mg}$$

The patient should receive Nebcin 100 mg q.8.h.

d. How many mL of Nebcin (80 mg/2 mL) should the patient receive q.8.h. to equal the prescribed dosage (100 mg)?

$$80 \text{ mg} : 2 \text{ mL} :: 100 \text{ mg} : X \text{ mL}$$

$$80 X = 200$$

$$X = 2.5 \text{ mL}$$

The nurse should administer 2.5 mL of Nebcin (80 mg/2 mL) q.8.h.

To prepare the correct dosage for administration, the nurse would use two vials of Nebcin (80 mg/2 mL). Two mL (80 mg) would be withdrawn from one vial and 0.5 mL (20 mg) would be withdrawn from the second vial for a total of 2.5 mL.

Note
The second vial may be labeled:

<table>
<tr><td colspan="2" align="center">60 mg/1.5 mL</td></tr>
<tr><td>Date</td><td align="right">Signature</td></tr>
</table>

Store drug in refrigerator to be used with next dose.

☐ Practice Problems

Directions
Use the proportion formula to calculate the correct amount of drug to administer to the patient.

1. Order: Lanoxin® (digoxin) 0.125 mg IM q.d.
   Available: Lanoxin ampule labeled 0.25 mg per 1 cc.

   How many cc of Lanoxin (0.25 mg/cc) should you administer?

2. Order: Norzine® (thiethylperazine maleate) 8 mg IM stat.
   Available: Norzine ampule labeled 10 mg/2 mL.

   Mark the correct volume on the syringe shown in Figure 7.5.

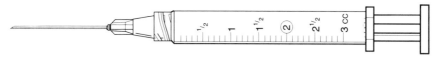

FIGURE 7.5.

3. Order: Hyper Hep® (hepatitis B immune globulin [human]) 0.06 mL/kg of body weight IM now.
   Patient weighs 99 lbs.
   Available: Vial labeled as shown in Figure 7.6.

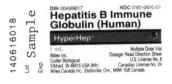

FIGURE 7.6.

How many mL of Hyper Hep should you administer?

4. Order: Pantopon® (hydrochloride of opium alkaloids) gr ⅙ IM q.4.h. PRN for pain.
   Available: Pantopon ampule containing ⅓ gr per 1 mL.

   How many mL of Pantopon (gr ⅓/mL) should the patient receive?

5. Order: Kantrex® (kanamycin sulfate) 0.75 g IM q.12.h.
   Available: Kantrex vial labeled 1.0 g per 3 mL.

   a. How many mL of Kantrex (1.0 g/3 mL) should you administer? Place the answer in the space provided in b.

   b. How many ♏ of Kantrex (0.75 g/＿＿＿ mL) should you administer?

6. Order: Enlon® (edrophonium chloride) gr ⅕ IM now.
   Available: Fifteen-mL multidose vial labeled Enlon 10 mg per/mL.

   Select the correct syringe (Fig. 7.7) and mark the volume you should administer.

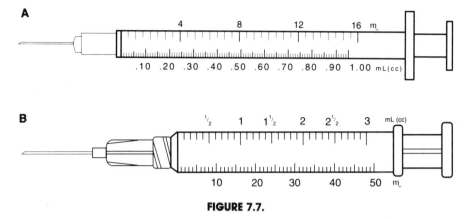

FIGURE 7.7.

7. Order: DDAVP® (desmorpressin acetate) 3 μg in two equally divided
   doses subc BID.
   Available: DDAVP ampule containing 4 μg/1 mL.

   a. How many μg of DDAVP should you administer per dose?

   b. How many mL of DDAVP (4 μg/mL) should you administer per
      each dose using a tuberculin syringe?

8. Order: Secobarbital Sodium (secobarbital sodium) gr ⅗ IM at 10 pm.
   Available: Single dose cartridge injector units with needle labeled
            Secobarbital gr ¾ per mL and gr 1½ per mL.

   a. Which cartridge injector unit of Secobarbital should you use? Place
      the strength/volume of the drug selected in the space provided in
      b.

   b. How many mL of Secobarbital (gr ____/____ mL) should you
      administer?

c. How many mL should you expel from the prefilled cartridge unit before administering the prescribed dose?

9. Order: Konakion® (phytonadione) 7.5 mg IM q.d.
   Available: Ampules of Konakion labeled 1 mg/0.5 mL and 10 mg/1 mL.

   a. Which ampule should you use?

   b. Mark the volume in minims that should be administered if either syringe is used (Fig. 7.8).

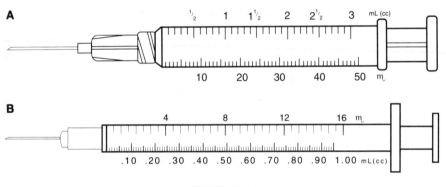

FIGURE 7.8.

10. Order: Neupogen® (filgrastim) 5 mcg/kg of body weight subcu. q.d.
    Patient's weight: 176 lbs.
    Available: Two vials labeled as shown in Figure 7.9.

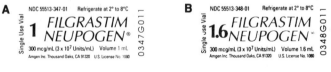

FIGURE 7.9.

a. How many mL of Neupogen should you administer?

b. Which vial will you use to prepare the ordered dose?

11. Order: Toradol® (ketorolac tromethamine) gr ½ IM @ 6 a.m., 2 p.m., and 10 p.m.
Available: Prefilled manufactured 1-mL syringes containing 15 mg/mL and 30 mg/mL and a 2-mL syringe containing 30 mg/mL.

a. Select the correct prefilled syringe and volume you should administer.

b. Your hospital is on military time. At what hours should the patient receive Toradol?

12. Order: Sandostatin® (octreotide acetate) 0.3 mg bid subcu.
Available: Multidose vial labeled Sandostatin 200 μg/mL.

Mark the volume that should be administered on the syringe shown in Figure 7.10.

1/2
1
1 1/2
2
2 1/2
3 cc

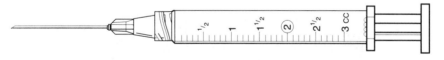

FIGURE 7.10.

13. Order: Aquasol A® (vitamin A palmitate) 35,000 U IM daily for 10 days.
Available: Vial labeled as shown in Figure 7.11.

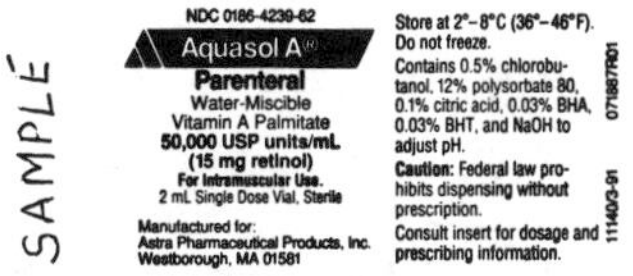
SAMPLE
NDC 0186-4239-62
Aquasol A®
Parenteral
Water-Miscible
Vitamin A Palmitate
50,000 USP units/mL
(15 mg retinol)
For Intramuscular Use.
2 mL Single Dose Vial, Sterile
Manufactured for:
Astra Pharmaceutical Products, Inc.
Westborough, MA 01581
Store at 2°–8°C (36°–46°F).
Do not freeze.
Contains 0.5% chlorobutanol, 12% polysorbate 80, 0.1% citric acid, 0.03% BHA, 0.03% BHT, and NaOH to adjust pH.
Caution: Federal law prohibits dispensing without prescription.
Consult insert for dosage and prescribing information.
071887R01
111403-91

FIGURE 7.11.

a. How many mL should you administer?

b. How many units of Aquasol are contained in the vial?

14. Order: Scopolamine Hydrobromide (scopolamine hydrobromide) gr $\frac{1}{200}$ IM at 7:30 a.m.
    Available: Single-dose vial containing Scopolamine Hydrobromide 400 mcg/mL.

    a. How many gr equal 400 mcg?

    b. How many mL of Scopolamine (_____ gr/mL) should you administer?

15. Order: Furosemide® (furosemide) 15 mg IM qd.
    Available: Vials labeled as shown in Figure 7.12.

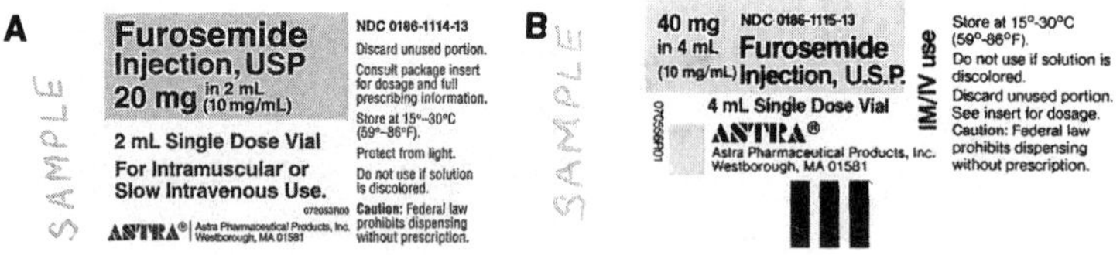

A

SAMPLE

Furosemide Injection, USP
20 mg in 2 mL (10 mg/mL)
2 mL Single Dose Vial
For Intramuscular or
Slow Intravenous Use.
ASTRA® | Astra Pharmaceutical Products, Inc. Westborough, MA 01581

NDC 0186-1114-13
Discard unused portion.
Consult package insert for dosage and full prescribing information.
Store at 15°–30°C (59°–86°F).
Protect from light.
Do not use if solution is discolored.
Caution: Federal law prohibits dispensing without prescription.

B

SAMPLE

40 mg NDC 0186-1115-13
in 4 mL **Furosemide**
(10 mg/mL) **Injection, U.S.P.**
4 mL Single Dose Vial
ASTRA®
Astra Pharmaceutical Products, Inc. Westborough, MA 01581

IM/IV use

Store at 15°–30°C (59°–86°F).
Do not use if solution is discolored.
Discard unused portion.
See insert for dosage.
Caution: Federal law prohibits dispensing without prescription.

FIGURE 7.12.

a. Which vial should you select?

b. On the syringe (Fig. 7.13) locate the amount of Furosemide you should administer.

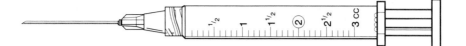

FIGURE 7.13.

16. Order: Versed® (midazolam HCl) 0.07 mg/kg IM @ 6 a.m.
    Available: 1-, 2-, and 5-mL vials labeled Versed 5 mg/mL.
    Patient's weight: 209 lbs.

    a. Identify vial you should use and the volume to be administered.

    b. Using military time, at what hour should the drug be administered?

17. Order: Hyper-TeT (tetanus immune globulin [human]) 225 units deep
    IM now.
    Available: 1-mL vial labeled as shown in Figure 7.14.

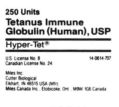

FIGURE 7.14.

Mark the volume you should administer on the syringe shown in Figure 7.15.

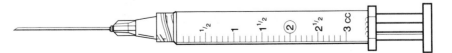

FIGURE 7.15.

18. Order: Nembutal® (pentobarbital sodium) gr iss IM q h.s.
Available: Nembutal vial labeled 2.5 Gm per 50 mL.

How many mL of Nembutal (2.5 Gm/50 mL) should you administer?

19. Order: Lupron® (leuprolide acetate) gr ⅟₆₀ subcu daily.
Available: A 2.8 mL multidose vial labeled Lupron 5 mg per 1 mL.

Mark the volume that should be administered on the syringe in Figure 7.16.

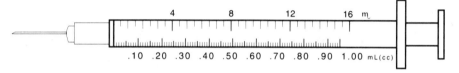

FIGURE 7.16.

20. Order: Calcimar® (calcitonin-salmon) 4 IU/kg IM @ 0600 and 1800 × 2 days, then increase to 6 IU/kg IM @ 0600 and 1800 on the third day.
Available: Calcimar 2 mL vial containing 200 IU/mL.
Patient's weight: 154 lbs.

a. How many mL should you administer to equal each dose the first two days; then the third day?

b. At what time frequency is the patient receiving Calcimar?

21. Order: Demerol® (meperidine hydrochloride) 60 mg and Phenergan® (promethazine hydrochloride) 25 mg IM at 6:30 a.m.
Available: Demerol ampule 100 mg/2 mL and Phenergan ampule 25 mg/1 mL.

a. How many mL of Demerol (100 mg/2 mL) should the patient receive?

b. Locate the amount of solution you will have in the syringe when you withdraw the Demerol, then locate the amount you will have when you add the Phenergan to the syringe (Fig. 7.17).

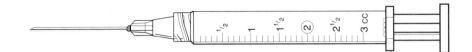

FIGURE 7.17.

Note

When preparing two medications in one syringe, first withdraw the fractional part of a medication or the medication contained in a multidose vial, then add the medication contained in an ampule. Measuring each medication in a specific syringe and then combining them in one syringe may be necessary to avoid contamination of a vial with the medication in the syringe. If one of the medications is contained in a prefilled syringe and the second in a multidose vial, it may be necessary to measure each medication separately, then combine to avoid contamination of the vial with the medication in the prefilled syringe.

22. Order: Morphine sulfate® (morphine sulfate) gr ⅙ IM q.6.h. p.r.n. for pain.
    Available: Morphine sulfate ampules labeled 5 mg/mL, 8 mg/mL, and 15 mg/mL.

    a. Which ampule of Morphine sulfate should you use?

    b. If you use the ampule of Morphine sulfate labeled 15 mg/mL, how many mL should you administer?

23. Order: Epogen® (epoetin alfa) 2400 U subcu Mondays, Wednesdays, and Fridays @ 5 p.m.
    Available: Single-use vial labeled as shown in Figure 7.18.

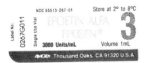

FIGURE 7.18.

a. Mark the correct amount you should administer on the syringe shown in Figure 7.19.

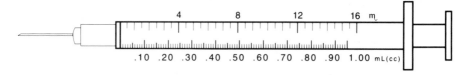

FIGURE 7.19.

b. Your hospital is on military time. At what hour will the patient receive the drug?

c. Literature states the usual dosage is 100 U/kg per day. This patient weighs 88 lbs. Is the patient receiving above, below, or the usual recommended dosage?

24. Order: Amikin® (amikacin sulfate) 0.45 Gm IM q.12.h.
    Available: Amikin vial labeled 500 mg/2 mL.
        The literature states that the recommended daily dosage of Amikin for adults is 15 mg per kg of body weight divided in two or three equal doses administered at equally divided intervals.
    Patient's weight: 132 lbs.

a. How many mg of Amikin has the physician ordered to be administered q.12.h.?

b. Is the prescribed dosage above, below, or the same as the recommended dosage?

c. How many mL of Amikin (500 mg/2 mL) should you administer to equal the prescribed dose?

25. Order: Bumex® (bumetamide) gr $\frac{1}{120}$ IM now.
    Available: Two-mL vial labeled Bumex 0.25 mg/mL.

    How many mL should you administer?

26. Order: Actimmune® (interferon gamma-1B) 1.5 mcg/kg body weight
    subcu on Mondays, Wednesdays, & Fridays at 0900.
    Available: Single-dose vial labeled Actimmune 100 mcg/0.5 mL.
    Patient's weight: 132 lbs.

    Mark the correct amount that should be administered on the syringe
    shown in Figure 7.20.

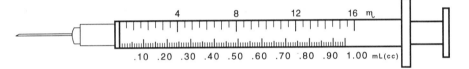

FIGURE 7.20.

27. Order: Stadol® (butorphanol tartrate) 1.5 mg and Phenergan (pro-
    methazine hydrochloride) 12.5 mg IM on call to surgery.
    Available: Single-dose vial containing Stadol 2 mg/mL and an ampule
    labeled Phenergan 25 mg/mL.

    a. How many ♏ of Stadol (2 mg/_____ ♏) and Phenergan (25 mg/
       _____ ♏) should you administer?

    b. Locate the amount of solution you will have in the syringe (Fig.
       7.21) when you withdraw the Stadol, then locate the amount you
       will have when you add the Phenergan to the syringe.

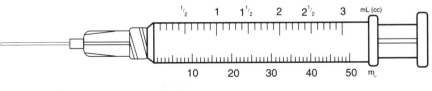

FIGURE 7.21.

c. How many total ℳ of Stadol and Phenergan will you have in the syringe?

28. Order: Bentyl® (dicyclomine hydrochloride) 0.08 g daily in 4 equally divided doses over 24 hours.
    Available: Ten-mL vial containing 100 mg of Bentyl.

    a. How many mL should the patient receive per dose?

    b. If the patient receives the first dose at 0600, when will the patient receive the next three doses?

29. Order: Tagamet® (cimetidine hydrochloride) 0.25 g q8h IM.
    Available: Multidose 8-mL vial labeled Tagamet 300 mg/2 mL.

    a. How many mL of Tagamet (_____ g/2 mL) should the patient receive?

    b. The vial of Tagamet contains a total of how many g of the drug?

    c. How many 0.25 g doses can you obtain from the 8-mL vial of Tagamet?

30. Order: Robinul® (glycopyrrolate injection) 0.12 mg, Stadol® (butor-

phanol tartrate) 0.5 mg, and Vistaril® (hydroxyzine hydrochloride) 20 mg IM on call for surgery.
Available: Single-dose 1-mL vial labeled Robinul 0.2 mg, unit dose
1-mL vial containing 50 mg of Vistaril, and Stadol 1-mL
vial containing 1 mg.

a. How many mL of each drug will you prepare to equal the dosages
   ordered?

Robinul

Stadol

Vistaril

b. Locate the amount of solution you will have in the syringe shown
   in Figure 7.22 when you withdraw the Stadol. Then locate the
   amount you will have when you add the Robinul. Finally, locate
   the amount you will have when you add the Vistaril.

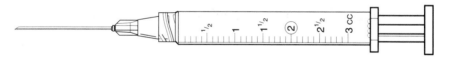

FIGURE 7.22.

☐ Answers

1. 0.25 mg : 1 cc :: 0.125 mg : X cc

$$0.25 \ X = 0.125$$

$$X = 0.5 \ cc$$

2. 10 mg : 2 mL :: 8 mg : X mL

$$10 X = 16$$

$$X = 1.6 \text{ mL}$$

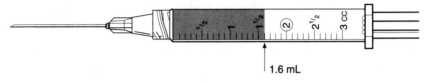

1.6 mL

FIGURE 7.23.

3. 2.2 lbs : 1 kg :: 99 lbs : X kg

$$2.2 X = 99$$

$$X = 45 \text{ kg}$$

0.06 mL : 1 kg :: X mL : 45 kg

$$1 X = 2.7 \text{ mL}$$

4. ⅓ gr : 1 mL :: ⅙ gr : X mL

$$⅓ X = ⅙$$

$$X = ½ \text{ mL or } 0.5 \text{ mL}$$

5. a. 1.0 g : 3 mL :: 0.75 g : X mL

$$1.0 X = 2.25$$

$$X = 2.25 \text{ mL}$$

  b. 1 mL : 16 ♏ :: 2.25 mL : X ♏

$$1 X = 36 ♏ \text{ or } ♏ \text{ xxxvi}$$

6. 1 gr : 60 mg :: ⅕ gr : X mg

$$1 X = {}^{60}\!/_5 = 12 \text{ mg}$$

10 mg : 1 mL :: 12 mg : X mL

$$10 X = 12$$

$$X = 1.2 \text{ mL}$$

When making conversions, choose the one which is easiest for you. You could have converted the available drug (10 mg) to grains (gr $\frac{1}{6}$).

gr $\frac{1}{6}$: 1 mL :: gr $\frac{1}{5}$: X mL

$\frac{1}{6}$ X = $\frac{1}{5}$

X = 1.2 mL

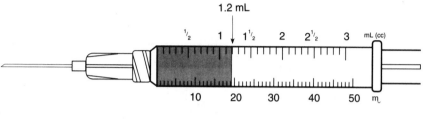

FIGURE 7.24.

Select the 3-mL syringe. The tuberculin syringe has a maximum volume of 1 mL.

7. a. 3 μg : 2 doses :: X μg : 1 dose

   2 X = 3

   X = 1.5 μg per dose

   b. 4 μg : 1 mL :: 1.5 μg : X mL

   4 X = 1.5

   X = 0.375 mL or 0.38 mL

8. a. Secobarbital injector unit labeled $\frac{3}{4}$ gr/mL to avoid waste.

   b. gr $\frac{3}{4}$: 1 mL :: gr $\frac{3}{5}$: X mL

   $\frac{3}{4}$ X = $\frac{3}{5}$

   X = $\frac{4}{5}$ mL or 0.8 mL

   c. 1.0 mL available
      $\underline{-0.8 \text{ mL dosage}}$
       0.2 mL expelled

9. a. 10 mg/1 mL ampule

   b. 10 mg : 16 ℳ :: 7.5 mg : X ℳ

   10 X = 120

   X = 12 ℳ

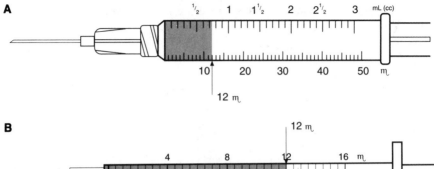

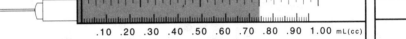

FIGURE 7.25.

10. a. 2.2 lbs : 1 kg :: 176 lbs : X kg

$$2.2 \, X = 176$$

$$X = 80 \text{ kg}$$

5 mcg : 1 kg :: X mcg : 80 kg

$$1 \, X = 400 \text{ mcg (dose ordered)}$$

300 mcg : 1 mL :: 400 mcg : X mL

$$300 \, X = 400$$

$$X = 1.33 \text{ mL or } 1.3 \text{ mL}$$

b. Use the vial that contains 1.6 mL to minimize waste.

11. a. 1 gr : 60 mg :: ½ gr : X mg

$$1 \, X = {}^{60}\!/_2 = 30 \text{ mg}$$

Select the 1-mL syringe containing 30 mg to minimize waste and reduce volume administered to the patient. Administer total contents (1 mL).

b. 0600, 1400, 2200

12. 1 mg : 1000 µg :: 0.3 mg : X µg

$$1 \, X = 300 \text{ µg}$$

200 µg : 1 mL :: 300 µg : X mL

$$200 \, X = 300$$

$$X = 1.5 \text{ mL}$$

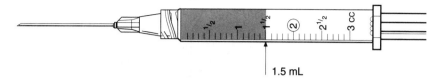

1.5 mL

FIGURE 7.26.

13. a. 50,000 U : 1 mL :: 35,000 U : X mL

$$50,000 \ X = 35,000$$

$$X = 0.7 \ mL$$

   b. 100,000 units

14. a. 1000 mcg : 1 mg :: 400 mcg : X mg

$$1000 \ X = 400$$

$$X = 0.4 \ mg$$

         1 mg : $\frac{1}{60}$ gr :: 0.4 ($\frac{4}{10}$) mg : X gr

$$1 \ X = \frac{1}{150} \ gr$$

  OR

     ($\frac{1}{60}$ gr = 1 mg = 1000 mcg)

   1000 mcg : $\frac{1}{60}$ gr :: 400 mcg : X gr

$$1000 \ X = \frac{400}{60}$$

$$X = \frac{1}{150} \ gr$$

  b. gr $\frac{1}{150}$: 1 mL :: gr $\frac{1}{200}$: X mL

$$\frac{1}{150} \ X = \frac{1}{200}$$

$$X = \frac{150}{200} \ or \ 0.75 \ mL$$

15. a. Vial containing 20 mg/2 mL to minimize waste. Label states to discard unused portion.

  b. 20 mg : 2 mL :: 15 mg : X mL

$$20 \ X = 30$$

$$X = 1.5 \ mL$$

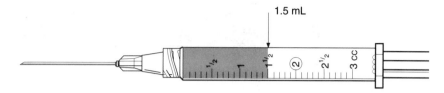

1.5 mL

FIGURE 7.27.

16. a. 2.2 lbs : 1 kg :: 209 lbs : X kg

   2.2 X = 209

   X = 95 kg

   0.07 mg : 1 kg :: X mg : 95 kg

   1 X = 6.65 mg (dose ordered)

   5 mg : 1 mL :: 6.65 mg : X mL

   5 X = 6.65

   X = 1.33 or 1.3 mL

   Select 2-mL vial

   b. 0600

17. 250 U : 1 mL :: 225 U : X mL

   250 X = 225

   X = 0.9 mL

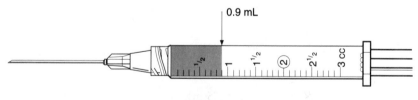

0.9 mL

FIGURE 7.28.

18. 15 gr : 1 Gm :: 1½ gr : X Gm

   15 X = 1½ (1.5)

   X = 0.1 Gm

OR

1 gr : 0.06 Gm :: 1.5 gr : X Gm

$$1 X = 0.09 \text{ Gm}$$

2.5 Gm : 50 mL :: 0.1 Gm : X mL

$$2.5 X = 5$$

$$X = 2 \text{ mL}$$

OR

2.5 Gm : 50 mL :: 0.09 Gm : X mL

$$2.5 X = 4.5$$

$$X = 1.8 \text{ mL}$$

19. 1 gr : 60 mg :: $\frac{1}{60}$ gr : X mg

$$X = \frac{60}{60} = 1 \text{ mg}$$

5 mg : 1 mL :: 1 mg : X mL

$$5 X = 1$$

$$X = 0.2 \text{ mL}$$

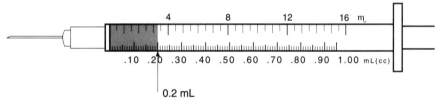

0.2 mL

FIGURE 7.29.

20. a. 2.2 lbs : 1 kg :: 154 lbs : X kg

$$2.2 X = 154$$

$$X = 70 \text{ kg}$$

4 IU : 1 kg :: X IU : 70 kg

$$1 X = 280 \text{ IU (dose ordered)}$$

200 IU : 1 mL :: 280 IU : X mL

$$200 X = 280$$

$$X = 1.4 \text{ mL (first 2 days)}$$

6 IU : 1 kg :: X IU : 70 kg

1 X = 420 IU (dose ordered 3rd day)

200 IU : 1 mL :: 420 IU : X mL

200 X = 420

X = 2.1 mL (3rd day)

b. q 12 h

21. a. 100 mg : 2 mL :: 60 mg : X mL

100 X = 120

X = 1.2 mL

b.

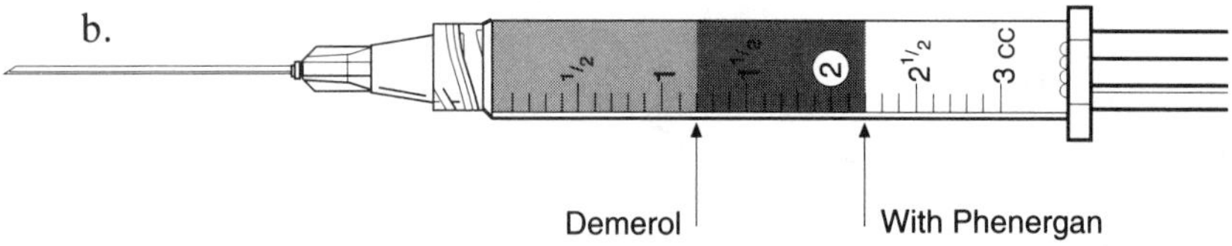

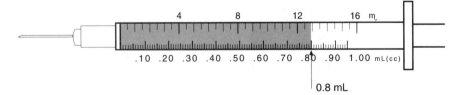

Demerol   With Phenergan

FIGURE 7.30.

22. a. 1 gr : 60 mg :: gr $\frac{1}{6}$: X mg

$1 X = \frac{60}{6}$

X = 10 mg

Preferably use the 15 mg/mL ampule for economical purposes, but any of the ampules could be used to prepare the correct dosage.

b. 15 mg : 1 mL :: 10 mg : X mL

15 X = 10

X = 0.67 mL

23. a. 3000 U : 1 mL :: 2400 U : X mL

3000 X = 2400

X = 0.8 mL

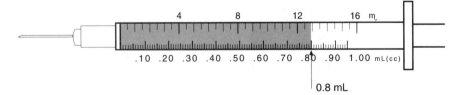

0.8 mL

FIGURE 7.31.

b. 1700

c. 2.2 lbs : 1 kg :: 88 lbs : X kg

      2.2 X = 88

         X = 40 kg

   100 U : 1 kg :: X U : 40 kg

     1 X = 4000 U

Receiving below the usual recommended dose.

24. a. 1000 mg : 1 Gm :: X mg : 0.45 Gm

       1 X = 450 mg

  b. 2.2 lbs : 1 kg :: 132 lbs : X kg

      2.2 X = 132

        X = 60 kg (pt. wt. in kg)

  15 mg : 1 kg :: X mg : 60 kg

    1 X = 900 mg (daily recommended dose)

Prescribed dosage (900 mg/day) is the same as the recommended dosage (900 mg/day).

  c. 500 mg : 2 mL :: 450 mg : X mL

      500 X = 900

        X = 1.8 mL

25. 1 gr : 60 mg :: $\frac{1}{120}$ gr : X mg

     1 X = $\frac{60}{120}$

      X = 0.5 mg

 0.25 mg : 1 mL :: 0.5 mg : X mL

    0.25 X = 0.5

      X = 2 mL

26. 2.2 lbs : 1 kg :: 132 lbs : X kg

     2.2 X = 132

       X = 60 kg

 1.5 mcg : 1 kg :: X mcg : 60 kg

    1 X = 90 mcg (dose ordered)

$$100 \text{ mcg} : 0.5 \text{ mL} :: 90 \text{ mcg} : X \text{ mL}$$
$$100 \text{ X} = 45$$
$$X = 0.45 \text{ mL}$$

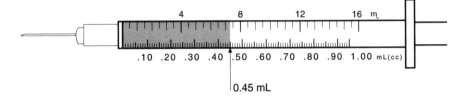

0.45 mL

FIGURE 7.32.

27. a. $2 \text{ mg} : 16 \text{ m} :: 1.5 \text{ mg} : X \text{ m}$

$$2 \text{ X} = 24$$
$$X = 12 \text{ m of Stadol}$$

$$25 \text{ mg} : 16 \text{ m} :: 12.5 \text{ mg} : X \text{ m}$$
$$25 \text{ X} = 200$$
$$X = 8 \text{ m of Phenergan}$$

b.

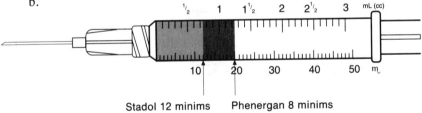

Stadol 12 minims   Phenergan 8 minims

FIGURE 7.33.

b.

c.   12 m Stadol
   + 8 m Phenergan
   20 m Total

28. a. $1 \text{ g} : 1000 \text{ mg} :: 0.08 \text{ g} : X \text{ mg}$

$$1 \text{ X} = 80 \text{ mg}$$

$$80 \text{ mg} : 4 \text{ doses} :: X \text{ mg} : 1 \text{ dose}$$
$$4 \text{ X} = 80$$
$$X = 20 \text{ mg (each dose)}$$

100 mg : 10 mL : : 20 mg : X mL

100 X = 200

X = 2 mL

b. 1200, 1800, 2400

29. a. 1000 mg : 1 g : : 300 mg : X g

1000 X = 300

X = 0.3 Gm

0.3 g : 2 mL : : 0.25 g : X mL

0.3 X = 0.5

X = 1.67 mL

b. 0.3 g : 2 mL : : X g : 8 mL

2 X = 2.4

X = 1.2 g

c. 0.25 g : 1 dose : : 1.2 g : X dose

0.25 X = 1.2

X = 4.8 doses

30. a. 0.2 mg : 1 mL : : 0.12 mg : X mL

0.2 X = 0.12

X = 0.6 mL of Robinul

1 mg : 1 mL : : 0.5 mg : X mL

1 X = 0.5 mL of Stadol

50 mg : 1 mL : : 20 mg : X mL

50 X = 20

X = 0.4 mL of Vistaril

b.

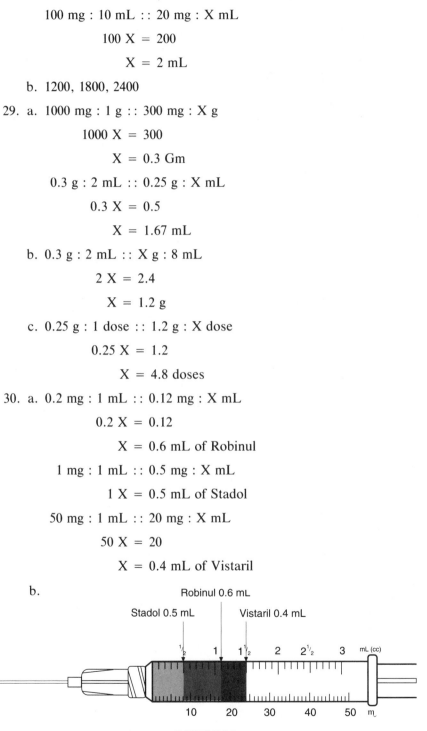

FIGURE 7.34.

Note

When preparing several medications in one syringe from vials, add the required volume of air to each vial before withdrawing medication. This will prevent possible contamination of the vials with medication and will facilitate easier preparation.

If you missed more than 5 problems, review the chapter and the problems before starting the next chapter.

Powder and Crystalline-Form Drugs | 8

Reconstitution of Drugs in Powder and Crystalline Form

Drugs that are unstable in solution are manufactured in crystalline or powder form. Prior to use, the dry medication must be dissolved or reconstituted (mixed with Sterile Water for Injection, Bacteriostatic Water for Injection, 0.9% Sodium Chloride Injection, or some other special solvent). The dry form of the drug is contained in sterile single dose vials or ampules or multidose vials. The specific type of solvent and the amount needed to dissolve the drug are stated in the directions for reconstitution provided by the manufacturer. This information may also be found in drug reference books.

Always read the directions carefully; vials of the same drug manufactured in different strengths may require different volumes of solvent. For example, the 0.5-Gm vial of Claforan® (cefotaxime sodium) requires a minimum of 2 mL of solvent for reconstitution. The 1.0-Gm vial of Claforan requires a minimum of 3 mL and the 2.0-Gm vial requires 5 mL of solvent.

Vials of the same drug may also require different volumes and types of diluent for different routes of administration. For example, the 2-g vial of Meslin (Fig. 8.1) requires 8 mL of sterile water for injection or 0.5% lidocaine HCl injection (without epinephrine) for reconstitution for IM use. For IV use, 20 mL of diluent is required.

The volume of diluent will also vary with how the drug is administered intravenously. For direct intravenous (bolus) use, the 1.0-Gm Tazicef® (ceftazidime) vial requires 3 mL of diluent. For administration by intravenous

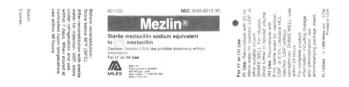

FIGURE 8.1.

infusion, the 1.0-Gm vial requires 10 mL of diluent plus an additional 90 mL of diluent prior to administration.

This chapter will focus on reconstitution of drugs for parenteral administration.

Displacement

In dry form, powders or crystals occupy a greater volume than after reconstitution. Once the powder or crystals are dissolved in the solvent, the volume may be more than the amount of solvent added. A manufacturer may tell you to "add 4.2 mL Sterile Water for Injection to a vial containing 1 Gm of drug in dry form." Once mixed, the vial contains 5 mL of the 1-Gm drug in solution, which is 0.8 mL more than you added. The difference in the amount of solvent and the reconstituted volume is called displacement. This drug occupies or displaces 0.8 mL in volume measurement (Fig. 8.2).

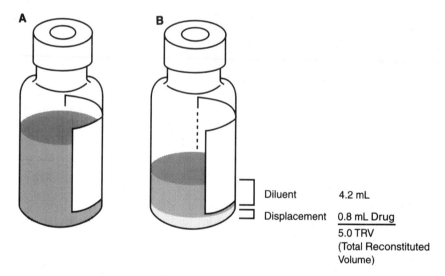

Diluent	4.2 mL
Displacement	0.8 mL Drug
	5.0 TRV
	(Total Reconstituted Volume)

FIGURE 8.2. A. Drug in dry form. **B.** Drug reconstituted.

The amount of displacement varies from drug to drug. The displacement may be so minute that the increased volume is not considered in calculating the prescribed dose. On the other hand, the total volume may be increased significantly (eg, 0.5 cc to 4 cc) and must be considered when calculating the prescribed dose.

After adding the appropriate amount of solvent, mix the drug by rolling the vial between the palms of your hands or by shaking the bottle. To ensure correct measurement do not withdraw the solution from the vial until it is free from bubbles and all the powder is dissolved.

Reconstituted multidose vials must be labeled by the nurse who prepares the drug. The label should contain:

- The date mixed.

- The date and time to discard the solution.*

- The dosage in a specific volume (eg, 100 mg/cc).

- The initials of the nurse who prepared the drug.

Other information that may be required on the label includes the type and amount of solvent added and how the solution should be stored. The label added to the container should not obscure the name of the drug. Never use a drug that has been reconstituted but has not been labeled.

Preparing Powder or Crystalline Drugs for Intramuscular or Subcutaneous Administration

When powder or crystalline drugs are prepared for administration, various situations may be encountered. Four common situations with example problems are described.

Situation 1

The dosage prescribed may be equivalent to the total strength of the drug contained in the vial or ampule. The drug company insert or flier may indicate a specific amount of solvent required to mix the drug or suggest various amounts of solvent that may be added to the vial. In preparing the drug, the nurse should use the volume of solvent that will prepare the *prescribed dosage* in:

- A concentration that will cause minimal tissue irritation, and

- A volume that can be correctly measured and safely administered by the intramuscular or subcutaneous route. The preferred volume is between 0.5 mL and 3 mL for IM administration. The preferred volume for the subcutaneous route should not exceed 1 to 1.5 mL.

Volumes not considered safe to inject in one site should be divided and administered in two sites.

---

* The length of time the reconstituted drug can be retained is defined in the manufacturers' directions.

Example 1

Order: Primaxin® (imipenem–eilastatin sodium) 750 mg IM NOW.
Available: Primaxin 750-mg vial. Dissolve in 3 mL of 1% lidocaine (without epinephrine) HCl solution.

a. How many mL of solvent should you add to the vial?

3 mL

b. What amount should you administer to equal the prescribed dosage?
Withdraw the *total* amount in the vial, which will equal 750 mg.

Example 2

Order: Cefobid® (cefoperazone) 1 Gm IM q.12.h.
Available: Cefobid 1-Gm vial. Add 2.6 mL of solvent to obtain a concentration of 333 mg/mL; add 3.8 mL to obtain a concentration of 250 mg/mL.

a. How many mL of solvent should you add to the vial?

2.6 mL

b. How much solution should you withdraw to administer to equal the prescribed dose?
Withdraw the total amount in the vial, which will equal 1.0 Gm. To add 3.8 mL would increase the amount of solution you would need to administer.

Situation 2

The drug information sheet may not indicate the total reconstituted volume after adding the appropriate solvent or may not indicate a portion of the drug in a specific volume (information needed to calculate the prescribed dose). Under these conditions, the safest method to determine the dosage is to:

1. Mix the solvent and dry form of the drug until dissolved.

2. Withdraw the total amount into a syringe.

3. Note the total volume (you may have added 2 cc and now have 2.1 cc).

4. Use the new volume to calculate the correct dosage.

Example 1

Order: Pentam® 300 (pentamidine isethionate) 150 mg IM q day.
Available: Pentam vial containing 300 mg. The directions state to add 3 mL of Sterile Water for Injection.

a. How many mL of solvent should you add to the vial?

3 mL

b. What amount should you administer to equal the prescribed dose?
   Withdraw the entire contents of the 300-mg vial into a syringe.
   Measure this amount and return one half of the volume to the vial
   and administer the remaining one-half volume (150 mg) to the patient.

Example 2

Order: Mandol® (cefamandole nafate) 250 mg IM q.12.h.
Available: Mandol 1-Gm vial. Each 1-Gm vial should be diluted with
      3 mL of solvent.

a. How would you determine the amount of Mandol to administer to
   equal the prescribed dosage?
   Withdraw the total reconstituted contents in a syringe. Measure
   the amount of total volume. Then calculate the prescribed dose
   from the available total reconstituted volume.

Situation 3

The drug information may define various volumes of solvent that can be
added to a vial to derive a specific dosage per milliliter(s). The reconstituted
volume will be greater than the volume of the solvent added. The nurse must
carefully read the dilution table to determine:

• The strength of the vial to be used.

• The recommended amount of solvent to add to derive the prescribed dosage in a specific volume.

Example

Available: A 10-mL vial containing 1 Gm of Capastat Sulfate® (capreo-
      mycin sulfate).
Dissolve with 0.9% Sodium Chloride Injection according to Table 8.1.

a. How many mL of solvent should you add to the vial to obtain a
   prescribed dosage of 250 mg?

3.3 mL

b. How many mL should you administer to equal the prescribed dosage
   of 250 mg?

1 mL

TABLE 8.1. Capastat Sulfate Dilution Table

Diluent[a] Added to 1-Gm Vial (mL)	Approximate Concentration (mg per 1 mL)
2.15	350
2.63	300
3.3	250
4.3	200

[a] The terms diluent and solvent are used interchangeably to refer to the liquid used to dissolve dry forms of drugs.

    c. If you added 3.3 mL of solvent, how would you label the vial to define the dosage in a specific volume?

$$250 \text{ mg}/1 \text{ mL}$$

    d. What is the total reconstituted volume in the vial?

$$\frac{\text{Prescribed}}{\text{Dosage}} : \frac{\text{Known}}{\text{Volume}} :: \frac{\text{Total Dosage}}{\text{In Vial}} : \frac{\text{Unknown}}{\text{Total Volume}}$$

$$250 \text{ mg} : 1 \text{ mL} :: 1000 \text{ mg} : \text{X mL}$$

$$250 \text{ X} = 1000$$

$$\text{X} = 4 \text{ mL}$$

    e. What is the volume of displacement?

$$\begin{array}{ll} 4.0 \text{ mL} & \text{Total Reconstituted Volume} \\ \underline{-3.3 \text{ mL}} & \underline{\text{Solvent}} \\ 0.7 \text{ mL} & \text{Displacement} \end{array}$$

Situation 4

The prescribed dosage in a specific volume may not be identified in the dilution directions. Using the suggested dosage per volume stated in the directions, the nurse can derive the volume of the prescribed dosage. Remember that the prescribed dosage should be prepared in a volume that can be accurately measured and that is safe for intramuscular administration.

Example 1

    Order: Ceptaz® (ceftazidime) 500 mg IM q 12 h.
    Available: Ceptaz 1-g vial. Add 3 mL of Bacteriostatic Water for Injection. Each mL equals 250 mg of Ceptaz.

$$250 \text{ mg} : 1 \text{ mL} :: 500 \text{ mg} : X \text{ mL}$$

$$250 \text{ X} = 500$$

$$X = 2 \text{ mL}$$

Add 3 mL of diluent to the 1-g vial. Once it has dissolved, withdraw 2 mL, which equals the prescribed dosage (500 mg).

Label the vial to define a specific dosage per volume: 500 mg/2 mL or 250 mg/mL.

Example 2

Order: Pipracil® (piperacillin sodium) 1.5 g IM stat.
Available: A 2-g vial of Pipracil. Each gram should be reconstituted with 2 mL of diluent to yield a concentration of 1 Gm/2.5 mL.

How many mL of solvent should you add to the 2 g vial of Pipracil?

$$4 \text{ mL}$$

How many mL should you administer to equal the prescribed dosage?

$$1 \text{ Gm} : 2.5 \text{ mL} :: 1.5 \text{ Gm} : X \text{ mL}$$

$$1 \text{ X} = 3.75 \text{ mL}$$

☐ Practice Problems

1. Order: Claforan® (cefotaxime sodium) 1 g q 12 h IM.
   Available: A 2-g vial of Claforan. Add 5 mL of diluent to yield an approximate concentration of 330 mg/mL.

   a. How many mL will you administer to equal the prescribed dose?

   b. What is the total reconstituted volume?

2. Order: Primaxin® I.M. (imipenem–cilastatin sodium) 0.5 g q 12 h deep IM.
   Available: Vial labeled as shown in Figure 8.3.

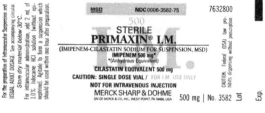

FIGURE 8.3.

a. How many mL of diluent should you add?

b. What solvent should you use?

c. How much volume do you administer to equal the dosage prescribed?

3. Order: Kefzol® (cefazolin sodium) 330 mg IM q.8.h.
   Available: 250 mg/10 mL and 1 Gm/10 mL vials of Kefzol.

   Reconstitute according to Table 8.2.

TABLE 8.2. Dilution Table for Kefzol® (Cefazolin Sodium, Lilly)

Vial Size	Diluent to Be Added (mL)	Approximate Available Volume (mL)	Approximate Average Concentration (mg/mL)
250 mg	2	2	125
500 mg	2	2.2	225
1 g[a]	2.5	3	330

[a] The 1-g vial should be reconstituted only with Sterile Water for Injection or Bacteriostatic Water for Injection.
Copyright © PHYSICIANS' DESK REFERENCE® 1993 edition. Published by Medical Economics Data, Montvale, NJ 07645. Reprinted by permission. All rights reserved.

a. What strength vial of Kefzol should you use?

b. How many mL of diluent should you add to the vial?

c. How many mL should you administer to equal the prescribed dosage?

d. What is the total reconstituted volume?

e. What is the displacement?

f. How should you label the vial to define the dosage per specific volume?

g. You reconstituted this vial November 1, at 9:00 A.M. When should the drug be discarded?

4. Order: Factrel® (gonadorelin hydrochloride) 0.1 mg subcu now.
   Available: Factrel 100-mcg and 500-mcg vials accompanied by an ampule containing 2 mL of a 2% benzyl alcohol in sterile water diluent. Reconstitute the 100-mcg vial with 1.0 mL of the diluent and the 500-mcg vial with 2.0 mL of the diluent. The unused reconstituted solution and diluent should be discarded.

a. Which vial will you prepare?

b. How many mL of diluent should you add to the vial?

c. How much volume should you administer to equal the prescribed dose?

5. Order: Cefotan® (cefotetan disodium) 1.5 g q 24 h IM.
   Available: A 2-g vial of Cefotan.
   Prepare the solution according to Table 8.3.

TABLE 8.3. Cefotan Dilution Table

For Intramuscular Use: Reconstitute with Sterile Water for Injection; Bacteriostatic Water for Injection; Normal Saline, USP; 0.5% Lidocaine HCl; or 1.0% Lidocaine HCl. Shake to dissolve and let stand until clear.

Vial Size	Amount of Diluent to Be Added (mL)	Approximate Withdrawable Vol. (mL)	Approximate Average Concentration (mg/mL)
1 gram	2	2.5	400
2 gram	3	4.0	500

a. How many mL of solvent should you add?

b. What types of solvent should you use?

c. How many mL should you administer to equal the prescribed dose?

d. What is the amount of displacement in the 2-g vial?

e. After withdrawing the prescribed dose, how many mg remain in the vial?

6. Order: Mezlin® (meziocillin sodium) 1.5 Gm q6h IM.
   Available: Mezlin 1-Gm vials. Dissolve in 3–4 mL of Sterile Water for Injection or 1% Lidocaine Hydrochloride Solution (without epinephrine).

   a. How many vials would you prepare for each dose?

   b. How many mL of solvent should you add to each vial?

   c. How would you prepare the amount of Mezlin needed to equal the prescribed dosage?

7. Order: Tazicef® (ceftazidime) 0.5 Gm IM q12h.
   Available: Tazicef 1-Gm and 2-Gm vials and a vial of Sterile Water for Injection.

   Reconstitute according to Table 8.4.

TABLE 8.4. Tazicef Reconstitution Table

Vial Size (Gm)	Diluent to Be Added (mL)	Approximate Available Volume (mL)	Approximate Average Concentration (mg/mL)
	Intramuscular or Intravenous Direct (Bolus) Injection		
1	3.0	3.6	280
	Intravenous Infusion		
1	10	10.6	95
2	10	11.2	180

Withdraw the total volume of solution into the syringe (the pressure in the vial may aid withdrawal). The withdrawn solution may contain some bubbles of carbon dioxide.

a. What strength Tazicef vial should you use?

b. How many mL of solvent should you add to the vial to prepare the prescribed dose?

c. How many mL should you administer to equal the prescribed dose of Tazicef?

d. How should you label the vial to define the dosage per specific volume?

8. Order: Kefzol® (cefazolin sodium) 500 mg IM q.12.h.
   Available: Vial labeled as shown in Figure 8.4.

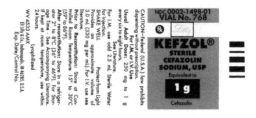

FIGURE 8.4.

a. What solvent should you use?

b. How many mL of diluent should you add to the vial?

c. How many mL should you administer to equal the prescribed dose?

d. What is the total reconstituted volume in this vial?

e. If the reconstituted vial is kept at room temperature, within how many hours should it be used?

9. Order: Ticar® (ticarcillin disodium) 60 mg/kg/day IM in equally divided doses q 8 h.
   Available: 1-Gm vial of Ticar. Reconstitute with 2 mL of diluent and use promptly. Each 2.6 mL of the reconstituted solution will contain 1 Gm of Ticar.
   Patient weighs 88 lbs.

   Locate the amount (Fig. 8.5) that you should administer q 8 h to equal the prescribed dosage.

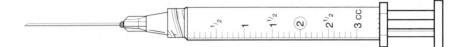

FIGURE 8.5.

10. Available: A 5,000,000-unit vial of Buffered Pfizerpen (penicillin G potassium).

TABLE 8.5. Buffered Pfizerpen Reconstitution Table

Desired Concentration (Units/mL)	Approximate Volume (mL) 1,000,000 Units	Solvent for Vial of 5,000,000 Units
50,000	20	—
100,000	10	—
250,000	4	18.2
500,000	1.8	8.2
750,000	—	4.8
1,000,000	—	3.2

Reconstitute according to Table 8.5. Use Table 8.5 to answer the following questions:

a. How many mL of diluent should you add to obtain a prescribed dosage of 750,000 units?

b. The physician prescribed a dosage of 500,000 units. How many mL of diluent should you add to the 5,000,000-unit vial to obtain the prescribed dose in 1 mL?

c. You reconstituted the 5,000,000-unit vial with 8.2 mL of diluent. How many mL of the reconstituted drug should you administer to equal a prescribed dosage of 750,000 units?

d. After adding 3.2 mL of diluent to the 5,000,000-unit vial, what is the total reconstituted volume?

11. Order: Zinacef® (cefuroxime sodium) 0.5 Gm IM q8h.
    Available: Zinacef vial to be reconstituted according to Table 8.6.

TABLE 8.6. Zinacef Dilution Table*a*

Strength	Amount of Diluent to Be Added (mL)	Volume to Be Withdrawn (mL)	Approximate Concentration (mg/mL)
750-mg vial	3.0 (IM)	Total	220
750-mg vial	8.0 (IV)	Total	90
1.5-g vial	16.0 (IV)	Total	90
750-mg infusion pack	100.0 (IV)	—	7.5
1.5-g infusion pack	100.0 (IV)	—	15

a Zinacef is a suspension at IM concentrations.
Copyright © PHYSICIANS' DESK REFERENCE® 1993 edition. Published by Medical Economics Data, Montvale, NJ 07645. Reprinted by permission. All rights reserved.

a. What strength Zinacef vial should you reconstitute?

b. How many mL of solvent should you add to the vial?

c. How many mL of Zinacef should you administer to equal the prescribed dosage?

d. What is the total reconstituted volume in this vial?

12. Order: Mefoxin® (cefoxin sodium) 1 g q 8 h IM.
    Available: Vial labeled as shown in Figure 8.6.

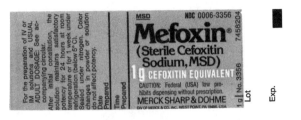

FIGURE 8.6.

The accompanying circular directs to reconstitute the 1-Gm vial with 2 mL of diluent and the 2-GM vial with 4 mL of diluent. Each mL will contain 400 mg of Mefoxin.

a. How many mL of diluent should you add to the available vial?

b. Identify the volume (Fig. 8.7) that you should administer to equal the dosage ordered.

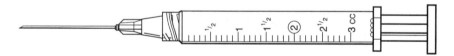

FIGURE 8.7.

c. What is the displacement volume?

13. Order: Azactam® (aztreonam) 400 mg q 12 h IM.
    Available: Azactam 500-mg single-use vial.
    Reconstitute with 3 mL of diluent per gram of aztreonam.

    Describe how you would prepare the Azactam to administer the correct dosage.

14. Order: Monocid® (cefonicid sodium) 750 mg IM daily.
    Available: Vial containing 1 g of Monocid and directions for reconstitution (Table 8.7).

TABLE 8.7. Monocid Reconstitution Table

Single-Dose Vials
For IM injection, IV direct (bolus) injection, or IV infusion, reconstitute with Sterile Water for Injection according to the following table. SHAKE WELL.

Vial Size	Diluent to Be Added	Approx. Avail. Volume	Approx. Avg. Concentration
500 mg	2.0 mL	2.2 mL	225 mg/mL
1 gram	2.5 mL	3.1 mL	325 mg/mL

These solutions of Monocid (sterile cefonicid sodium, SK&F) are stable 24 hours at room temperature or 72 hours if refrigerated (5°C.). Slight yellowing does not affect potency.

a. What kind of diluent and how many mL should you add to the available vial?

b. Using Figure 8.8, locate the amount you should administer.

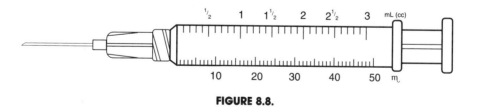

FIGURE 8.8.

c. What is the amount of displacement in the 0.5-g vial? in the 1-g vial?

15. Order: Cefizox® (ceftizoxime sodium) 250 mg IM q.12.h.
    Available: Vials of Cefizox labeled 1 Gm and 2 Gm.
    Following reconstitution, Cefizox is stable 48 hrs if refrigerated. Use
    Table 8.8 to answer the questions that follow.

TABLE 8.8. Cefizox Dilution Table

Preparation of Parenteral Solution			

RECONSTITUTION
IM Administration: Reconstitute with Sterile Water for Injection. SHAKE WELL.

Vial Size (Gm)	Diluent to Be Added (mL)	Approximate Available Volume (mL)	Approximate Average Concentration (mg/mL)
1	3.0	3.7	270
2ª	6.0	7.4	270

ª When administering 2-Gm IM doses, the dose should be divided and given in different large muscle masses.

IV Administration: Reconstitute with Sterile Water for Injection. SHAKE WELL.

Vial Size (Gm)	Diluent to Be Added (mL)	Approximate Available Volume (mL)	Approximate Average Concentration (mg/mL)
1	10	10.7	95
2	20	21.4	95

a. Which vial should you reconstitute?

b. How many mL of diluent should you add to the vial?

c. How many mL of Cefizox should you administer?

   d. You reconstituted this vial December 1 at 10 A.M. When should
      the drug be discarded?

16. Order: Fortaz® (ceftazidine) 250 mg q 12 h IM.
    Available: A 0.5-g vial of Fortaz.
    Follow Table 8.9 to answer the questions that follow:

TABLE 8.9. Preparation of Fortaz Solutions

Size	Amount of Diluent to be Added (mL)	Approximate Available Volume (mL)	Approximate Ceftazidime Concentration (mg/mL)
Intramuscular			
500-mg vial	1.5	1.8	280
1-gram vial	3.0	3.6	280
Intravenous			
500-mg vial	5.0	5.3	100
1-gram vial	10.0	10.6	100
2-gram vial	10.0	11.5	170
Infusion Pack			
1-gram vial	100[a]	100	10
2-gram vial	100[a]	100	20
Pharmacy Bulk Package			
6-gram vial	26	30	200

[a] *Note:* Addition should be in two stages (see Instructions for Constitution accompanying the product package insert).
Copyright © PHYSICIANS' DESK REFERENCE® 1993 edition. Published by Medical Economics Data, Montvale, NJ 07645. Reprinted by permission. All rights reserved.

   a. How many mL of diluent should you add to this vial?

   b. Locate on Figure 8.9 the volume in minims that should be admin-
      istered to equal the prescribed dose.

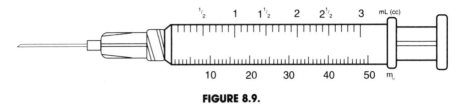

FIGURE 8.9.

c. What is the total reconstituted volume in this vial?

17. Order: Cefobid® (cefoperazone sodium) 1.5 Gm IM q12h from a reconstituted vial yielding a 250 mg/mL concentration.
Available: Cefobid 2-Gm vial.
Reconstitute the vial with Sterile Water for Injection and 2% Lidocaine Hydrochloride Injection (Table 8.10).

TABLE 8.10. Cefobid Dilution Table

	Final Cefoperazone Concentration (mg/mL)	Step 1 Volume of Sterile Water (mL)	Step 2 Volume of 2% Lidocaine (mL)	Withdrawable Volume (mL)[a,b]
1-Gm vial	333	2.0	0.6	3
	250	2.8	1.0	4
2-Gm vial	333	3.8	1.2	6
	250	5.4	1.8	8

When a diluent other than Lidocaine HCl Injection (USP) is used, reconstitute as
follows:

	Cefoperazone Concentration (mg/mL)	Volume of Diluent to Be Added (mL)	Withdrawable Volume (mL)[a]
1-Gm vial	333	2.6	3
	250	3.8	4
2-Gm vial	333	5.0	6
	250	7.2	8

[a] There is sufficient excess present to allow for withdrawal of the stated volume.
[b] Final lidocaine concentration will approximate that obtained if a 0.5% Lidocaine Hydrochloride Solution
is used as diluent.

a. Which solvent should you add first to the vial?

b. How many mL of Sterile Water for Injection should you add to the vial?

c. After dissolving the powder in the first solvent, how many mL of 2% Lidocaine Hydrochloride Injection would you add to the vial?

d. How many mL of Cefobid equal the prescribed dose?

e. How would you prepare the amount of Cefobid needed to administer to the patient?

f. What is the amount of displacement in the 2-Gm vial?

18. Order: Protropin® (somatrem for injection) 0.05 mg/kg IM three times a week.
    Available: Protropin 5-mg and 10-mg vials.
    Reconstitute 5-mg vial with 1–5 mL of the accompanying diluent.
    Reconstitute the 10-g vial with 1–10 mL of the diluent.
    Patient's weight: 110 lbs.

a. How many mg equals the prescribed dosage?

b. Describe how you will prepare the vial and the amount you will administer to equal the prescribed dose.

☐ **Answers**

1. a. 330 mg : 1 mL : : 1000 mg : X mL

           330 X = 1000

              X = 3.03 or 3 mL

   b. 330 mg : 1 mL : : 2000 mg : X mL

           330 X = 2000

              X = 6.06 or 6 mL

2. a. 2 mL

   b. 1% lidocaine HCl without epinephrine

   c. After agitating (mixing the diluent and powder) the vial, withdraw and administer the total contents, which equal 500 mg.

3. a. 1 Gm

   b. 2.5 mL

   c. 1 mL

   d. 330 mg : 1 mL : : 1000 mg : X mL

           330 X = 1000

              X = 3.03 or 3 mL

   e.   3.0 mL Total Reconstituted Volume

      −2.5 mL Diluent

        0.5 mL Displacement

   f. 330 mg/1 mL

   g. November 2, at 9 A.M.

4. a. 1000 mcg : 1 mg : : X mcg : 0.1 mg

           1 X = 100 mcg

   Select the 100-mcg vial

   b. 1 mL

   c. Total amount of reconstituted solution in the vial, which equals 0.1 mg Factrel.

5. a. 3 mL

   b. Sterile Water for Injection
   Bacteriostatic Water for Injection

Normal Saline
0.5% Lidocaine HCl
1% Lidocaine HCl

c. 500 mg : 1 mL : : 1500 mg : X mL

$$500 \, X = 1500$$

$$X = 3 \text{ mL}$$

d.   4.0 mL Total Reconstituted Volume

$\underline{-3.0 \text{ mL}\ \text{ Diluent}}$

    1.0 mL Displacement

e.   2000 mg

$\underline{-1500 \text{ mg}}$

    500 mg Remain

6. a. 2 vials

   b. 3 mL (always use the smallest amount)

   c. Withdraw total volume. Measure the amount and retain ½ of the volume in the syringe (0.5 Gm); then withdraw the total volume (1.0 Gm) from the other vial. Because the total volume exceeds 4.5 mL, divide the volume in 2 syringes and administer 2 injections.

7. a. 1-Gm vial

   b. 3 mL

   c. 0.280 Gm : 1 mL : : 0.5 Gm : X mL

$$0.280 \, X = 0.5$$

$$X = 1.78 \text{ or } 1.8 \text{ mL}$$

   d. 0.5 Gm/1.8 mL

8. a. Sterile Water for Injection

   b. 2.5 mL

   c. 330 mg : 1 mL : : 500 mg : X mL

$$330 \, X = 500$$

$$X = 1.5 \text{ mL}$$

   d. 3 mL

   e. 24 hours

9. 2.2 lbs : 1 kg : : 88 lbs : X kg

$$2.2 \, X = 88$$

$$X = 40 \text{ kg}$$

60 mg : 1 kg :: X mg : 40 kg

1 X = 2400 mg (dosage per day)

3 doses : 2400 mg :: 1 dose : X mg

3 X = 2400

X = 800 mg (each dose q8h)

1000 mg : 2.6 mL :: 800 mg : X mL

1000 X = 2080

X = 2.08 or 2.1 mL

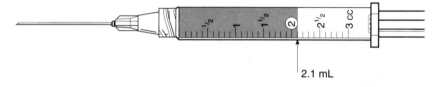

2.1 mL

FIGURE 8.10.

10. a. 4.8 mL

b. 8.2 mL

c. 500,000 U : 1 mL :: 750,000 : X mL

500,000 X = 750,000

X = 1.5 mL

d. 1,000,000 U : 1 mL :: 5,000,000 U : X mL

1,000,000 X = 5,000,000

X = 5 mL TRV

11. a. 750-mg vial

b. 3 mL

c. 0.220 Gm : 1 mL :: 0.5 Gm : X mL

0.220 X = 0.5

X = 2.27 or 2.3 mL

d. 220 mg : 1 mL :: 750 mg : X mL

220 X = 750

X = 3.4 mL

12. a. 2 mL

b. 400 mg : 1 mL :: 1000 mg : X mL

$$400 \text{ X} = 1000$$

$$\text{X} = 2.5 \text{ mL}$$

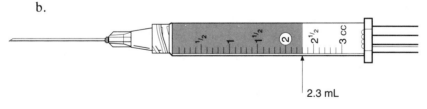

2.5 mL

FIGURE 8.11.

c. 2.5 mL − 2.0 mL = 0.5 mL

13. Add 1.5 mL of diluent to the 500-mg vial. Withdraw total contents into syringe to determine total reconstituted volume. Calculate correct dose. For example, if the total reconstituted volume is 1.6 mL, you would administer 1.3 mL.

$$500 \text{ mg} : 1.6 \text{ mL} :: 400 \text{ mg} : \text{X mL}$$

$$500 \text{ X} = 640$$

$$\text{X} = 1.28 \text{ or } 1.3 \text{ mL}$$

14. a. Sterile Water for Injection—2.5 mL diluent

b.

2.3 mL

FIGURE 8.12.

$$325 \text{ mg} : 1 \text{ mL} :: 750 \text{ mg} : \text{X mL}$$

$$325 \text{ X} = 750$$

$$\text{X} = 2.31 \text{ mL}$$

c.   2.2 mL TRV (total reconstituted volume)
   −2.0 mL Diluent
   0.2 mL Displacement in 0.5-g vial

OR

   3.1 mL TRV
  −2.5 mL Diluent
   0.6 mL Displacement in 1-g vial

15. a. 1-Gm vial to prevent waste due to loss of stability

   b. 3.0 mL

   c. 270 mg : 1 mL :: 250 mg : X mL

$$270 \text{ X} = 250$$
$$\text{X} = 0.93 \text{ or } 0.9 \text{ mL}$$

   d. December 3 at 10 A.M.

16. a. 1.5 mL

   b.

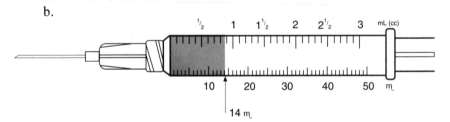

FIGURE 8.13.

280 mg : 16 ♏ :: 250 mg : X ♏
$$280 \text{ X} = 4000$$
$$\text{X} = 14.28 \text{ or } 14 \text{ ♏}$$

   c. 1.8 mL

17. a. Sterile Water for Injection

   b. 5.4 mL

   c. 1.8 mL

   d. 2 Gm : 8 mL :: 1.5 Gm : X mL

$$2 \text{ X} = 12$$
$$\text{X} = 6 \text{ mL}$$

   e. Divide the amount equally in 2 syringes

   f.   5.4 mL Sterile Water
         1.8 mL 2% Lidocaine
         7.2 mL Total Solvent

          8.0 mL Total Reconstituted Volume
       −7.2 mL Solvent
          0.8 mL Displacement

18. a. 2.2 lbs : 1 kg :: 110 lbs : X kg

$$2.2 \text{ X} = 110$$

$$\text{X} = 50 \text{ kg}$$

    0.05 mg : 1 kg :: X mg : 50 kg

$$1 \text{ X} = 2.5 \text{ mg}$$

   b. Select 5-mg vial, add 2 mL of diluent, and withdraw to determine total volume. Administer half of the total volume to equal the 2.5-mg prescribed dose.

Insulin

Insulin, a hormone normally produced by the pancreas, is essential for the metabolism of blood sugar and for the maintenance of proper blood sugar level. Inadequate secretion of insulin leads to improper metabolism of carbohydrates and fats and brings on the characteristics of hyperglycemia (high blood sugar) and glycosuria (glucose in the urine) associated with diabetes mellitus. Individuals with these symptoms may need to supplement the body with injections of insulin on a regular basis to sustain life.

Bottled insulin, used for replacement therapy, is obtained from animal and human sources. Beef and pork pancreas have been the main source of insulin for many years. Human insulin does not come directly from human beings but is made to be like the insulin produced by the human body. Human insulin is derived one of two ways: Recombinant DNA technology derives a synthetic insulin from *Escherichia coli* or by a process that chemically alters pork insulin to make human insulin. Technology has provided us with a purer, more predictable, and more readily available form of the hormone.

The standard of measure for insulin is the unit. Most insulin is dispensed in bottles containing 10 milliliters of 100 insulin units per milliliter (U-100) or a total of 1000 available units of insulin. Insulin concentrations are also available in U-40 (40 units per milliliter) and U-500 (500 units per milliliter) but are rarely used. A small amount of U-40 insulin is sold in the United States. U-500 is only used in an extreme situation in a controlled setting.

Two companies (Lilly and Novo Nordisk) manufacture over 40 different types of insulin distributed in the United States. The type of insulin tells you how fast the particular insulin starts to work and how long it works. Insulin has a rapid, intermediate, or long action. Table 9.1 provides a sample of the wide variety of insulins available.

The physician usually orders insulin by **source or species** (animal or human), **type** (Regular, NPH, Lente, and so forth), and **concentration** (U-100), as well as the specific **amount** and **time** to be administered. Many physicians will not necessarily specify the concentration, because U-100 is considered ''generic.'' The brand name (manufacturer) may be specified if the physician has a preference. It is important to ask the patient what specific kind of insulin they have been taking at home, because a change in brand name (manufacturer), type (Regular, NPH, Lente), source (beef, pork, beef/

TABLE 9.1. Varieties of Insulin[a]

Type	Manufacturer	Source	Strength
Rapid-acting (Onset 0.5–4 hours, duration 6–16 hours)			
Iletin II (Regular)	Lilly	Beef*	U-100
Iletin II (Regular)	Lilly	Pork	U-100, U-500
Semilente	Novo Nordisk	Beef	U-100
Velosulin Human (Regular)	Novo Nordisk	Human	U-100
Humulin R (Regular)	Lilly	Human	U-100
Novolin R (Regular)	Novo Nordisk	Human	U-100
Iletin I (Regular)	Lilly	Beef/Pork*	U-40, U-100
Intermediate-acting (Onset 1–4 hours, duration 24 hours)			
Humulin L	Lilly	Human	U-100
Insulatard NPH Human	Novo Nordisk	Human	U-100
Novolin N	Novo Nordisk	Human	U-100
Iletin II Lente	Lilly	Beef*	U-100
Iletin II NPH	Lilly	Pork	U-100
Lente Purified Pork	Novo Nordisk	Pork	U-100
Lente Insulin	Novo Nordisk	Beef	U-100
Semilente Iletin I	Lilly	Beef/Pork*	U-40, U-100
Mixtures (Onset 0.5–2 hours, duration 24 hours)			
Mixtard (30% Regular, 70% NPH)	Novo Nordisk	Pork	U-100
Mixtard Human 70/30	Novo Nordisk	Human	U-100
Humulin 70/30	Lilly	Human	U-100
Humulin 50/50	Lilly	Human	U-100
Long-acting (Onset 4–6 hours, duration 36 hours)			
Iletin II PZI	Lilly	Beef	U-100
Ultralente	Novo Nordisk	Beef	U-100
Iletin I PZI	Lilly	Beef/Pork	U-100
Humulin U (Ultralente)	Lilly	Human	U-100

[a] This is only a sample of the varieties of insulins available. For a more complete list consult drug references.
* Effective September 1, 1993, Eli Lilly and Company discontinued some of their beef and beef/pork insulins.

pork, or human), and/or method of manufacture (recombinant DNA versus animal-source insulin) might result in an unpredicted response or a need for a change in dosage.

Sample Order

Source	Type	Concentration	Dose	Route	Time
Humulin	L	U-100	16 units	sq	q am

In this order the patient is to receive 16 units of U-100 (100 units per cc) concentration Humulin (human) L (Lente; intermediate acting) insulin subcutaneously each morning. You would determine the specific time to allow administration approximately one-half hour before the morning meal.

Sample Order

Type	Dose	Route	Time
NPH	30 U	SC	ac q am

This order would need clarification with the patient and physician. The source needs to be clarified. Has the patient been receiving beef (Iletin II NPH), pork (Insulatard NPH), beef/pork (Iletin I NPH), or human (Humulin N or Novolin N) insulin? Remember U-100 is considered generic unless specified.

Sample Order

Dose	Type	Dose	Type
10 units of	Regular Insulin and	15 units of	NPH q am

This order requires the mixing of two different types of insulin. It is important NOT to mix sources. You would need to clarify if the physician preferred human or one of the other forms of insulin. In addition, you would need to find out what the person had used in the past. The route is not specified, but when insulins are combined they should only be administered subcutaneously. **Regular insulin can be given intravenously.**

Preparing Insulin for Injection

After validation of the order, the next step in prepreparing insulin for injection is to check the manufacturer's label on the bottle to ensure that you have an exact match between order and product. Figure 9.1 presents an example of the information that needs to be checked.

Insulin is measured in unique units and should be measured in a syringe calibrated to match the concentration of the insulin. Insulin syringes are manufactured by several companies, and they are available in 100 U/1 cc, 50 U/0.5 cc, 30 U/0.3 cc, and 25 U/0.25 cc for use with U-100 insulin (Fig. 9.2).

When using U-100 insulin you should use a U-100 calibrated syringe (100 units per cc). Figure 9.3 shows two types of U-100 1-cc syringes. One (Fig. 9.3A) is calibrated in single unit markings and one (Fig. 9.3B) in increments of two units per marking. The one with single units has odd num-

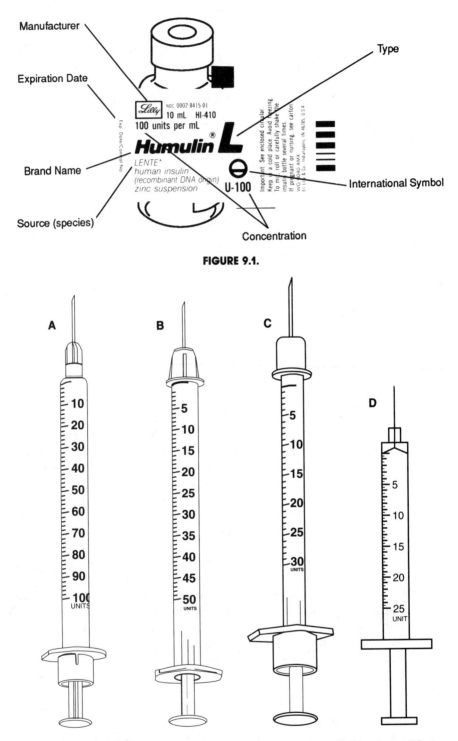

FIGURE 9.1.

FIGURE 9.2. A variety of U-100 syringes. **A.** 100 units per cc. **B.** 50 units per 0.5 cc. **C.** 30 units per 0.3 cc. **D.** 25 units per 0.25 cc.

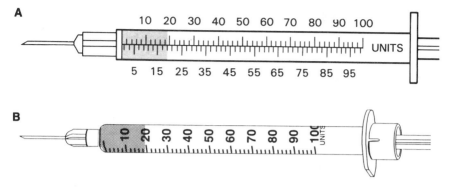

FIGURE 9.3. Two syringes containing 19 units of Novolin L U-100 insulin. **A.** Measured in single units. **B.** Measured in double units.

bers on one side and even numbers on the other side. To check the dosage you must turn the syringe slightly from side to side. This can make it a little difficult to see the precise dose. The syringe calibrated in twos makes it difficult to measure an odd number of units such as 19.

The "Lo-Dose" syringe helps solve the problem of measuring doses of less than 50, 30, or 25 units. They are calibrated in single units and the scale is enlarged and easier to read for patients with vision problems and health providers preparing injections. Figure 9.4 compares the same 19-unit dose

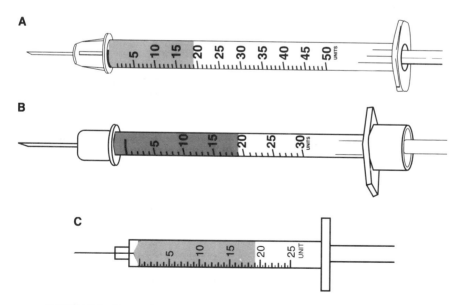

FIGURE 9.4. Comparison of dosage for Lo-Dose syringe. **A.** 0.5-cc (50-unit) U-100 syringe with 19 units of insulin. **B.** 0.3-cc (30-unit) U-100 syringe with 19 units of insulin. **C.** 0.25-cc (25-unit) U-100 syringe with 19 units of insulin.

measured in the various syringes. Remember that the concentration of the insulin is still 100 units per milliliter, so that the 50-U syringe is 50 U/0.5 cc, the 30-U syringe is 30 U/0.3 cc, and the 25-U syringe is 25 U/0.25 cc.

Tuberculin Syringe

Although the safest and most accurate way to measure insulin is to use an insulin syringe, it may become necessary to use the tuberculin syringe (TB) in an emergency. The tuberculin syringe substitution should only be used in the hospital situation.

Note
> The tuberculin syringe is 1 cc in volume and calibrated in hundredths. This makes using the TB syringe with U-100 insulin (100 U/cc) very easy.

Order: 15 units of U-100 Regular insulin subq now.
Available: U-100 Regular insulin and a TB syringe.
How many mL should you give?

CALCULATE DOSE

$$100 \text{ units} : 1 \text{ mL} :: 15 \text{ units} : X \text{ mL}$$

$$100 X = 15$$

$$X = 0.15 \text{ mL of U-100 Regular insulin}$$

The TB syringe is also calibrated in minims (Fig. 9.5). It has been the accepted practice to calculate insulin dose in minims if an insulin syringe was not available. The following examples are presented to help explain why the conversion to minims is no longer recommended.

TO CHANGE 0.15 CCs TO MINIMS

$$16 \; \text{m} : 1 \text{ mL} :: X \; \text{m} : 0.15 \text{ cc}$$

$$1 X = 2.4 \; \text{m}$$

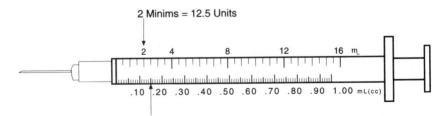

FIGURE 9.5.

If you follow the usual rules for rounding, the 2.4 minims would be 2 minims. Note on the syringe in Figure 9.5 that minims are measured in increments of 0.5, so 0.4 cannot be measured. If you gave 2 minims you would not be giving the correct dose.

$$16 \text{ m} : 100 \text{ units} :: 2 \text{ m} : X \text{ units}$$

$$16 \, X = 200$$

$$X = 12.5 \text{ units (order 15 units)}$$

This may seem like a small difference, but insulin dosage is increased or decreased by 1- or 2-unit intervals and a change in dosage due to miscalculation could interfere with the control of the disease.

One more example to stress the importance of calculating insulin in hundredths in the absence of the insulin syringe.

Order: 42 units Novolin N U-100 q am.

TO CONVERT TO MINIMS

$$100 \text{ U} : 16 \text{ m} :: 42 \text{ U} : X \text{ m}$$

$$100 \, X = 672$$

$$X = 6.7 \text{ minims}$$

If you round this to 7 minims, you will be giving too much insulin.

$$100 \text{ U} : 16 \text{ m} :: X \text{ U} : 7 \text{ m}$$

$$X = 43.75 \text{ or almost 44 units (42 U ordered)}$$

Note the difference in the amounts expressed in minims and hundredths on the syringe in Figure 9.6.

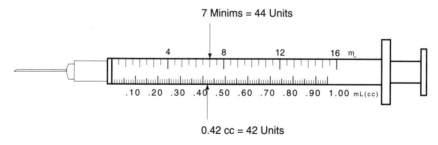

7 Minims = 44 Units

0.42 cc = 42 Units

FIGURE 9.6.

Always select the method of administration that will give you the most accurate dosage.

Figure 9.7 shows an example of what would happen if you had used a standard 3-cc syringe to measure the 42 units of insulin. Look at how small the volume (0.42 cc or 6.7 minims) would be in such a large syringe. Since

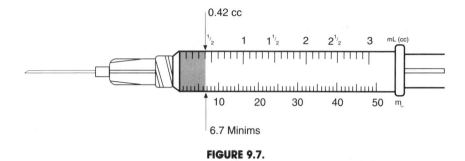

FIGURE 9.7.

the needle is detachable once the plunger is depressed, most of the insulin would still remain in the hub of the syringe, not in the patient. *Use of any syringe other than the appropriate insulin syringe or a tuberculin syringe is unsafe practice.*

Mixing Insulins

When mixing insulin, such as a short-acting and intermediate-acting insulin, always make sure that the insulins are made by the same manufacturer and are from the same source. Recent research reported by the American Diabetes Association suggests that Humulin N, R, and NPH can be mixed without any clinical differences in the action of the insulin. Semilente, Ultralente, and Lente may be combined, but mixtures of Human Lente and Regular insulin are subject to a binding phenomenon immediately upon mixing that delays the onset of regular insulin, reduces the peak activity, and prolongs the total duration. It may be necessary to give two injections if the individual uses Lente and Regular Humulin. Individuals who have achieved control although they mix them at home are advised to maintain their standardized administration procedure so as not to change the action of the medication.*

When mixing insulins in the same syringe, the regular insulin is always drawn first, and then the intermediate- or long-acting insulin. Make sure that you add the two together correctly so that you will have the correct amount. Figure 9.8 is an example of mixing two insulins in a syringe.

Any insulins that are mixed in the same syringe should be administered as quickly as possible to reduce any chance of change in concentration. If unsure about combining any insulins, consult with your pharmacist or other reference sources for more detailed explanation of the procedure.

---

* Anderson JH: New research—New ways for day to day diabetes care. *Med News* **8:**1–4, 1988.

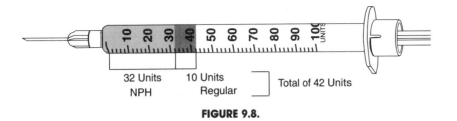

32 Units   10 Units

NPH   Regular   Total of 42 Units

FIGURE 9.8.

Preparing Insulin Based on Blood Sugar Tests

It is not uncommon for the physician to want the patient with diabetes to have regular insulin throughout the day. Infections and stress can increase the body's need for insulin. The most common method used to determine the dosage of insulin is the use of a sliding scale. The patient's serum glucose level is checked before meals, at bedtime, or at other designated intervals. If the serum glucose level is outside the normal range (70–110 mg/dL), the nurse or patient prepares the insulin dose according to a scale written by the physician. The sliding scale is different for each patient and is a part of the medication order. Regular insulin is always used with a sliding scale.

Here is an example of a sliding scale using serum blood glucose results.

Order: Blood Glucose by fingerstick a.c. and h.s. U-100 Regular insulin a.c. and h.s. according to Sliding Scale.

Sliding Scale

Blood Sugar (mg/dL)	Regular Insulin
↓ 150	0
151–200	2 units
201–240	4 units
241–280	6 units
281–330	8 units
↑ 330	call physician

At 1100 Judy's blood sugar was 235. Based on the scale the nurse would administer 4 units of U-100 Regular in a U-100 syringe (probably a U-100 Lo-Dose syringe). By 1630 her blood sugar was 145; the nurse told Judy she would receive no insulin before her evening meal.

☐ Practice Problems

1. Order: 35 units of Humulin N subq a.c. q am.
   Available: Humulin N U-100 and several insulin syringes.

a. What is the prescribed dose?

b. Which of the syringes shown in Figure 9.9 would allow you to prepare the most accurate dose?

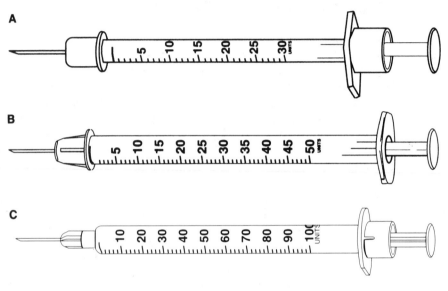

FIGURE 9.9.

c. On the syringe you selected, shade in the amount of of insulin you should administer.

2. Order: 55 units of Humulin L U-100 subq 0800 daily.
   Available: Humulin L U-100.

   a. What is the prescribed dose?

   b. Which syringe should you use?

c. How many units would you draw up in the syringe?

3. Your patient has been taking 20 units of Humulin R each morning before breakfast. The physician ordered her to have 20 units of Regular Insulin ac each am. Assume that the labels shown in Figure 9.10 are for the bottles available in your floor stock of insulin.

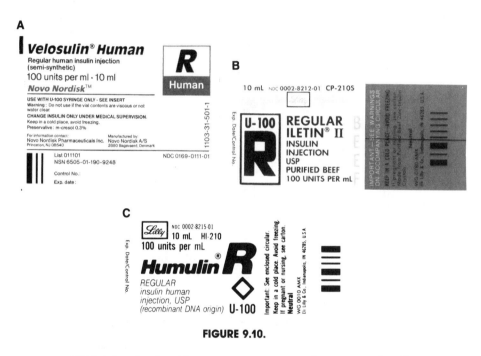

FIGURE 9.10.

a. Which bottle should you use to prepare the correct dose?

b. On the syringe in Figure 9.11, indicate how much you should administer.

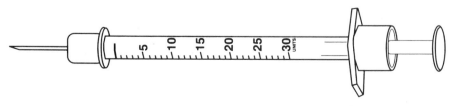

FIGURE 9.11.

4. Order: 15 units of Humulin R and 30 units of Humulin N subq q am.
   Available: Humulin R U-100 and Humulin N U-100.

   a. Which of the insulins should you draw into the syringe first?

   b. Mark the correct dosage on the syringe shown in Figure 9.12 (be
      sure to indicate which is R and which is N).

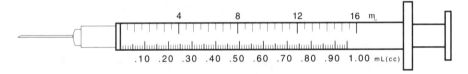

FIGURE 9.12.

5. Order: 45 units Novolin L U-100 subq daily.
   Available: U-100 Novolin L and a tuberculin syringe.

   a. How many units of insulin should you prepare?

   b. Mark the correct dosage on the syringe shown in Figure 9.13, using
      the mL scale.

FIGURE 9.13.

6. Your patient has the following sliding scale ordered.

Sliding Scale

Blood Sugar (mg/dL)	Regular Insulin
↓ 120	0
121–180	2 units
181–240	6 units
241–300	10 units
301–360	12 units
↑ 360	call doctor

Blood sugars by finger stick have been ordered ac and hs.
Order: 22 units of Novolin N q d at 0730, regular insulin by sliding
scale ac and hs.
Available: Those insulins with labels shown in Figure 9.14.

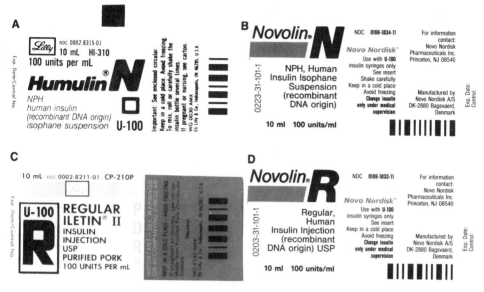

FIGURE 9.14.

At 0730 the blood sugar was 230 mg/dL.

a. What is the total number of units of insulin the patient should
receive?

b. What insulins should you combine?

At 1200 the blood sugar was 190 mg/dL.

c. On the syringe shown in Figure 9.15, indicate the amount of insulin
you should administer.

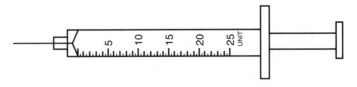

FIGURE 9.15.

At 1830 the blood sugar was 145 mg/dL.

d. How much insulin should the patient receive?

At 2200 the blood sugar was 118 mg/dL.

e. How much insulin should the patient receive?

f. How many total units of insulin did the patient receive during the day?

7. Order: 36 units of Mixtard 70/30 subq q am.
   Available: The insulins with labels shown in Figure 9.16.

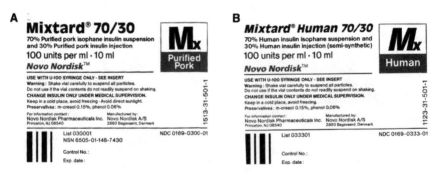

FIGURE 9.16.

a. Which one should you select? Why?

b. On the syringe shown in Figure 9.17, indicate the amount you should prepare for administration.

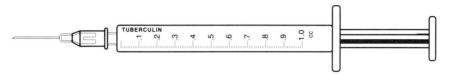

FIGURE 9.17.

8. Order: 56 units of Humulin N subq daily divided into two equal doses given at 7:30 am and 5:30 pm. Humulin R according to blood glucose results ac and hs.
   Available: Humulin N and R U-100 insulins.

Sliding Scale

Blood Sugar (mg/dL)	Regular Insulin
↓ 120	0
121–180	2 units
181–240	6 units
241–300	10 units
301–360	12 units
↑ 360	call doctor

For each of the times listed below, indicate the amount of insulin to be prepared for administration.

a. 7:30 am blood glucose 250 mg/dL.

b. On the syringe shown in Figure 9.18, indicate how much of each insulin you should prepare.

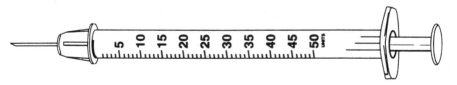

FIGURE 9.18.

c. 11:30 am blood glucose 136 mg/dL.

d. 5:30 pm blood glucose 215 mg/dL.

e. 11:00 pm blood glucose 118 mg/dL.

f. What was the total amount of insulin (Humulin N & R) for the day?

9. Order: 26 units of Ultralente U-100 subq daily.
   Available: U-100 Ultralente and a tuberculin syringe.
   How many mL should you administer?

10. Order: Insulin U-100 Regular by blood glucose results—ac and hs.

Sliding Scale

Blood Sugar (mg/dL)	Regular Insulin
↓ 120	0
121–180	2 units
181–240	6 units
241–300	10 units
301–360	12 units
↑ 360	call doctor

a. At 4:30 p.m. your patient's blood sugar was 200 mg. How many units of insulin should he receive?

b. Central Supply has not brought your insulin syringes—you must calculate using a TB syringe. How many hundredths of a cc should you administer? Mark the syringe shown in Figure 9.19 with the amount.

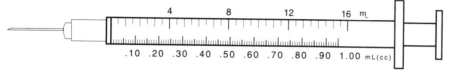

FIGURE 9.19.

☐ Answers

1. a. 35 units
   b. Select the 50 U/0.5 cc syringe—it is calibrated in single units.
   c.

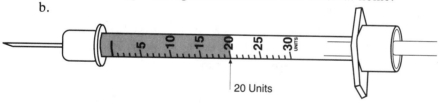

35 Units

FIGURE 9.20.

2. a. 55 units
   b. U-100 per 1 cc
      You will have to approximate the 55 units as the syringe is measured in twos. The closest measure is 54 or 56 units.

3. a. You should choose Humulin R shown in Figure 9.10C, because that is the type of Regular Insulin she had taken at home.
   b.

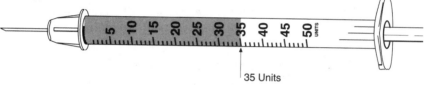

20 Units

FIGURE 9.21.

4. a. Always draw the Regular Insulin into the syringe first.
   b.

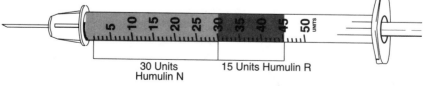

30 Units   15 Units Humulin R
Humulin N

FIGURE 9.22.

5. a. 45 units
   b.

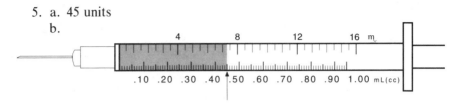

4. a. Always draw the Regular Insulin into the syringe first.
   b.
5. a. 45 units
   b.
6. a. 22 units of Novolin N plus 6 units of Regular = 28 units
   b. Follow the rules and use insulin manufactured by the same company and from the same source. You should use Novolin N, shown in Figure 9.14B, and Novolin R, shown in Figure 9.14D; they are both made by the same company and are of human source.
   c.

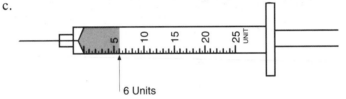

6 Units

FIGURE 9.24.

You should have marked 6 units. Check the sliding scale.
   d. 2 units
   e. None
   f. Total of 36 units—22 Novolin N and 14 Regular
7. a. Select Mixtard 70/30, shown in Figure 9.16A. The order said only 70/30; it did not specify Human.
   b.

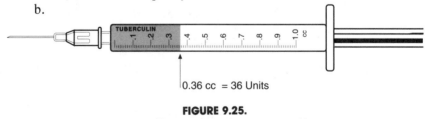

0.36 cc = 36 Units

FIGURE 9.25.

You should have drawn up 0.36 cc
8. a. 28 units of Humulin N and 10 units of Humulin R = 38 units.

b.

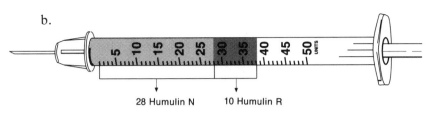

28 Humulin N   10 Humulin R

FIGURE 9.26.

c. 2 units of Humulin R
d. 6 units of Humulin R for blood sugar of 215 and 28 units of Humulin N = 34 units.
e. None for a blood sugar of 118
f. 56 units of Humulin N and 18 units of Humulin R = 74 total units for the day.
9. 0.26 cc measured in a tuberculin syringe.
10. a. 6 units
b. Administer 0.06 mL

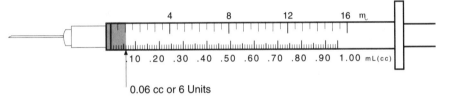

0.06 cc or 6 Units

FIGURE 9.27.

Intravenous Fluids and Medications | 10

Administration of intravenous fluids is common practice in a variety of health care settings, critical care, nonacute clinical units, and extended or home health care. The intravenous route is often preferred over the intramuscular route for antibiotics and pain medications. The method of IV medication administration varies. Medications may be added to large-volume IV fluid containers (1000 cc D5W with 40 mEq KCl to run 8 hours) and regulated for continuous infusion. Medications may also be added to small-volume containers (50–100 cc bag or bottle or Burette-style container) for administration on an intermittent basis through a heparin lock or as a secondary infusion through a primary IV line (Geopen 2 Gm in 50 ml D5W IVPB over 20 minutes). This is called IV Piggyback. Another form of intermittent infusion requires that the medication be injected directly into the bloodstream, IV push, either through a heparin lock, the port on the IV tubing, the port on a central line catheter, or directly into the vein (Lasix® 40 mg IV push now).

Hospital policies and physician's orders should indicate the infusion time and the amount of the dilution. If any of the information is not indicated in the order or policies, it is the responsibility of the nurse to contact the pharmacy and/or consult current pharmacology literature for this information.

Because fluids are going directly into the circulatory system, regulation of intravenous fluids is a critical nursing skill. It is essential that the patient not receive too much or too little IV fluid or medication.

To administer the prescribed fluid and/or medications, the nurse may be required to prepare the medication and add it to the fluids, to determine if the dose being administered is a safe dose, to calculate how much (mg, mcg, units) of a particular drug the patient is receiving at the current rate of fluid administration, and to determine the specific rate of flow and regulate, monitor, and maintain the flow rate.

The specific IV fluids and additives along with the infusion time are ordered by the physician (1000 cc D5W q8h or 1000 cc NS @ 125 mL/hr). The nurse will use the electronic or manual regulating equipment to monitor the infusion. The type of equipment used will determine the kind of calculating the nurse must do.

Calculating Flow Rate for Electronic Intravenous Flow Regulators

Health care institutions are increasing their use of electronic infusion devices to assist in IV management. When very small amounts of fluid or medication need to be infused over an extended time, the electronic device is ideal. There are many kinds of devices that function on gravity or pressure to maintain the flow rate and alarm when the infusion is interrupted. The operation of the equipment is beyond the scope of this text, but to use these devices the nurse must be able to calculate the volume per hour to program into the machine.

When the electronic flow regulator is used the physician usually orders the flow rate in milliliters (cc) per hour or specifies the amount of time to infuse the drug.

Example 1

Order: 1000 cc D5W IV over 8 hours.
Determine how many cc per hour this corresponds to. You can use your basic ratio and proportion method to determine the answer.

$$1000 \text{ cc} : 8 \text{ hours} :: X \text{ cc} : 1 \text{ hour}$$
$$8 X = 1000$$
$$X = 125 \text{ cc/h}$$

You would set the device to deliver 125 cc/h.

Example 2

Order: Ampicillin 500 mg in 100 mL D5W IVPB q8h. Run in 30 minutes.
Set the device at _____ mL/h.
The ratio and proportion method will also work easily.

$$100 \text{ mL} : 30 \text{ minutes} :: X \text{ mL} : 1 \text{ hour (60 minutes)}$$
$$30 X = 6000$$
$$X = 200 \text{ mL}$$

You would set the device to deliver 200 mL/h, and after 30 minutes the 100 mL would have been infused.

☐ Practice Problems

Calculate the flow rate (mL/h) you would program into the electronic flow regulator for the following amounts and time.

Amount (mL)	Time	mL/h
1. 1500	24 hours	
2. 1000	15 hours	
3. 1000	10 hours	
4. 600	3 hours	
5. 2000	24 hours	
6. 100	45 minutes	
7. 50	10 minutes	
8. 75	45 minutes	
9. 50	30 minutes	
10. 30	15 minutes	

☐ **Answers**

1. 1500 mL : 24 hours : : X mL : 1 hour

$$24 X = 1500$$
$$X = 62.5 \text{ or } 63 \text{ mL/h}$$

2. 1000 mL : 15 hours : : X mL : 1 hour

$$15 X = 1000$$
$$X = 66.6 \text{ or } 67 \text{ mL/h}$$

3. 1000 mL : 10 hours : : X mL : 1 hour

$$10 X = 1000$$
$$X = 100 \text{ mL/h}$$

4. 600 mL : 3 hours : : X mL : 1 hour

$$3 X = 600$$
$$X = 200 \text{ mL/h}$$

5. 2000 mL : 24 hours : : X mL : 1 hour

$$24 X = 2000$$
$$X = 83.33 \text{ or } 83 \text{ mL/h}$$

6. 100 mL : 45 minutes : : X mL : 60 minutes

$$45 X = 6000$$
$$X = 133.33 \text{ or } 133 \text{ mL/h}$$

7. 50 mL : 10 minutes : : X mL : 60 minutes

$$10 \text{ X} = 3000$$

$$\text{X} = 300 \text{ mL/h}$$

8. 75 mL : 45 minutes : : X mL : 60 minutes

$$45 \text{ X} = 4500$$

$$\text{X} = 100 \text{ mL/h}$$

9. 50 mL : 30 minutes : : X mL : 60 minutes

$$30 \text{ X} = 3000$$

$$\text{X} = 100 \text{ mL/h}$$

10. 30 mL : 15 minutes : : X mL : 60 minutes

$$15 \text{ X} = 1800$$

$$\text{X} = 120 \text{ mL/h}$$

Calculating Flow Rates for Manual Intravenous Regulators

Intravenous Drop Factors

Intravenous fluids are infused through plastic tubing attached at one end to the bag or bottle of fluid/medication and at the other end to a needle/catheter inserted into a blood vessel. Each administration set has a chamber with either a MACRO or MICRO dropper. The MACRO drop set will deliver either 10, 15, or 20 drops per milliliter depending on the manufacturer (Table 10.1) while the MICRO drop set, regardless of manufacturer, always delivers 60 drops per milliliter. Figure 10.1 shows an example of the MACRO and MICRO drop administration sets. It is not possible to tell the difference in the MACRO drop sets without looking at the packaging, while the MICRO drop is distinguished by the ''needle-like'' structure that protrudes into the drip chamber. To prevent errors in calculating infusion times, always check the manufacturers label to verify the drop rate of the administration set.

TABLE 10.1. Types of Intravenous Administration Sets

Manufacturer	Drops per Milliliter
Baxter—Travenol	10 and 60
Abbott	15 and 60
McGaw Cutter	20 and 60

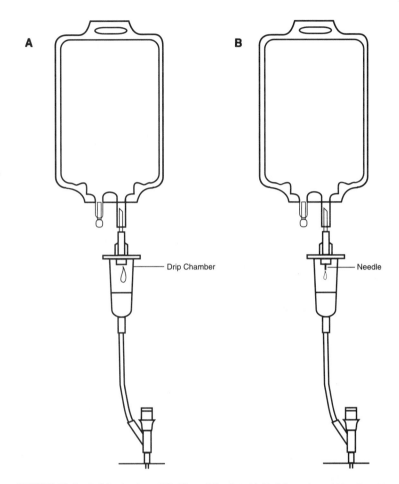

FIGURE 10.1. A. Macrodrop (10, 15, or 20 gtts/mL). **B.** Microdrop (60 gtts/mL).

Volume-controlled Administration Sets

When there is a need to protect the patient from receiving excess fluid, as with an infant who has a narrow fluid range or an adult kidney patient on fluid restriction, the volume-controlled set can be used (Fig. 10.2). It may be referred to as a pedi-drip, Buretrol, Soluset, or Volutrol. They are all very similar in shape and have a fluid chamber that will hold 100 to 150 mL of fluid. The drop factor is 60 gtts/mL.

These types of administration sets require the nurse to manually regulate the flow of fluid. First, the drop rate (drops per minute) must be calculated and then the flow set by adjusting a roller clamp or a screw clamp on the IV tubing. As the clamp is tightened, the internal diameter of the tubing is

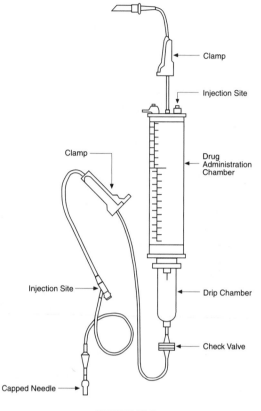

FIGURE 10.2.

decreased, and the rate of flow or drops per minute is decreased. The reverse is true as the clamp or screw is opened. The nurse times the drops using a watch that displays seconds or has a second hand and monitors the infusion frequently to ensure that the fluid is infused on time. A change in the position of the patient's arm could slow or increase the rate of flow; a kink in the tubing could also slow or stop the flow.

Flow rate can be calculated by a step-by-step method or a formula method.

Step-by-step Method

a. mL/h $\dfrac{\text{total mL fluid to be given}}{\text{hours to run}} = \text{mL/h}$

b. mL/min $\dfrac{\text{milliliter per hour}}{60 \text{ minutes}} = \text{mL/min}$

c. gtts/min $\text{mL/min} \times \text{drop per mL} = \text{gtt/min}$

Note

Carry calculations to 2 decimal places. Round gtts/min to the nearest whole number. You can only count whole drops.

Example 1 (macrodrop; 10, 15, or 20 drops/mL)

Order: 1000 cc D_5W IV to run 8 hrs.
Administration set delivers 10 drops/mL.
The IV should be regulated to deliver how many drops per minute?

a. $\dfrac{1000 \text{ cc}}{8 \text{ hours}} = 125$ cc/h

b. $\dfrac{125 \text{ cc/h}}{60 \text{ minutes}} = 2.1$ mL/min

c. 2.1 mL/min $\times$ 10 drops/mL = 21 drops/min

Example 2 (microdrop; 60 drops/mL)

Order: 500 cc D5RL IV to run 12 hours.
Administration set: microdrop (60 gtts/cc).
The IV should be regulated to deliver how many drops per minute?

a. $\dfrac{500 \text{ cc}}{12 \text{ hours}} = 41.66$ or 42 cc/h

b. $\dfrac{42 \text{ cc/h}}{60 \text{ minutes}} = 0.7$ cc/min

c. 0.7 cc/min $\times$ 60 drops/cc = 42 gtts/min

Note

When using a microdrop or pediatric administration set, the cc/hour are the same as the drops/min. Remembering this could save you some time.

Example 3

Many drugs that are administered intermittently are ordered to be infused in less than 1 hour. This enables you to begin with step b.

Order: Mandol® (cefamandole) 1 Gm q6h IVPB.
Available: Mandol 1 Gm in 50 cc NS.
The manufacturer recommends an infusion time of 30 minutes.
Administration set: 15 gtts/cc.

b. $\dfrac{50 \text{ cc}}{30 \text{ minutes}} = 1.666$ or 1.7 cc/min

c. 1.7 mL/min $\times$ 15 gtts/mL = 25.5 or 26 gtts/min

The above method is a logical step-by-step process that requires no memorization of a formula. Just think through the process of obtaining (1) cc/h, (2) cc/min, and (3) drops/min.

If you are comfortable with formulas, the three steps for determining the infusion rate can be combined into one formula. Use the computation that is easiest for you and allows for the least chance of error.

Formulas may also be used to calculate flow rate.

Formula I Method

This formula is recommended when the time prescribed for the infusion is in complete hours (2 hours, 6 hours, 8 hours, and so forth).

$$\frac{\text{amount of solution}}{\text{time in hours}} \times \frac{\text{drop factor}}{\text{60 minutes*}} = \text{drops/min}$$

Example 4

Order: 3000 cc of D5NS over the next 24 hours.
Administration set: 15 gtts/cc.
What is the drop rate?

$$\frac{3000 \text{ cc}}{24 \text{ hours}} \times \frac{15 \text{ gtt/cc}}{60 \text{ min/h}} = 31.25 \text{ or } 31 \text{ gtts/min}$$

If the infusion is to be administered in a portion of an hour, such as 1 hour 20 minutes or 30 minutes, the time must be converted into the decimal form 1.33 hours or 0.5 hours.

Example 5

Order: Bactrim® (trimethoprim and sulfamethoxazole) 500 mg IV in 150 cc D5W.
Administer in 90 minutes.
Administration set: 10 gtts/mL.
What is the drop rate?

$$\frac{150 \text{ cc}}{1.5 \text{ hours}} \times \frac{10 \text{ gtts/mL}}{60 \text{ minutes}} = 16.6 \text{ or } 17 \text{ gtts/min}$$

Remembering to change the minutes to the decimal form can be difficult for some people. Formula II may be helpful.

---

* This is a constant (60 min/h) and is inserted in the formula each time.

Formula II Method

This formula is recommended when the infusion time is one hour or less and the time can be easily converted into minutes.

$$\frac{\text{amount of solution}}{\text{time in minutes}} \times \text{drop factor} = \text{drops/min}$$

Example 6

Order: Aldomet® (methyldopa) 250 mg IVPB in 100 cc D5W.
Administer in 45 minutes.
Administration set: 10 gtts/cc.
What is the drop rate?

$$\frac{100 \text{ cc}}{45 \text{ minutes}} \times 10 \text{ gtt/cc} = 22.22 \text{ or } 22 \text{ gtts/min}$$

Some individuals may wish to use this formula exclusively, but remember when converting 6 hours to minutes (360) the number is large and this can cause some problems with math. Keep it simple and use the method that is best suited for your particular type of thinking.

☐ **Practice Problems**

Solve the following problems using the step-by-step method and the two formulas. Work them different ways so you will be able to decide which method is best for you.

	Amount (cc)	Time	Drop Factor	Gtt/min
1.	100	30 minutes	10	
2.	50	20 minutes	15	
3.	1000	8 hours	20	
4.	500	6 hours	15	

	Amount (cc)	Time	Drop Factor	Gtt/min
5.	250	3 hours	10	
6.	3000	12 hours	10	
7.	150	4 hours	60	
8.	125	60 minutes	15	
9.	1000	6 hours	20	
10.	30	1 hour	60	
11.	50	40 minutes	15	
12.	750	4 hours	10	
13.	100	45 minutes	20	
14.	50	15 minutes	10	

	Amount (cc)	Time	Drop Factor	Gtt/min
15.	50	1½ hours	60	
16.	500	3½ hours	10	
17.	20	20 minutes	15	
18.	400	6 hours	60	
19.	175	1½ hours	20	
20.	150	45 minutes	15	

☐ Answers

The answers to this section have been worked with one of the methods described in the text.

1. $\dfrac{100 \text{ cc}}{30 \text{ minutes}} \times 10 \text{ gtt/mL} = 33 \text{ gtts/min}$

2. $\dfrac{50 \text{ cc}}{20 \text{ minutes}} \times 15 \text{ gtts/mL} = 38 \text{ gtts/min}$

3. $\dfrac{1000 \text{ cc}}{8 \text{ hours}} \times \dfrac{20 \text{ gtts/mL}}{60 \text{ minutes}} = 42 \text{ gtts/min}$

4. $\dfrac{500 \text{ cc}}{6 \text{ hours}} \times \dfrac{15 \text{ gtts/mL}}{60 \text{ minutes}} = 21 \text{ gtts/min}$

5. $\dfrac{250 \text{ cc}}{3 \text{ hours}} \times \dfrac{10 \text{ gtts/mL}}{60 \text{ minutes}} = 14 \text{ gtts/min}$

6. $\dfrac{3000 \text{ cc}}{12 \text{ hours}} = 250 \text{ cc/h}$

$\dfrac{250 \text{ cc/h}}{60 \text{ minutes}} = 4.16 \text{ or } 4.2 \text{ cc/min}$

$4.2 \text{ cc/min} \times 10 \text{ gtts/mL} = 42 \text{ gtts/min}$

7. $\dfrac{150 \text{ cc}}{4 \text{ hours}} \times \dfrac{60 \text{ gtts/mL}}{60 \text{ minutes}} = 38 \text{ gtts/min}$

8. $\dfrac{125 \text{ cc}}{60 \text{ minutes}} \times 15 \text{ gtts/mL} = 31 \text{ gtts/min}$

9. $\dfrac{1000 \text{ cc}}{6 \text{ hours}} \times \dfrac{20 \text{ gtts/mL}}{60 \text{ minutes}} = 56 \text{ gtts/min}$

10. $\dfrac{30 \text{ mL}}{1 \text{ hour}} \times \dfrac{60 \text{ gtts/mL}}{60 \text{ minutes}} = 30 \text{ gtts/min}$

Remember cc/h = gtts/min when using 60 gtts/mL.

11. $\dfrac{50 \text{ mL}}{40 \text{ minutes}} \times 15 \text{ gtts/mL} = 19 \text{ gtts/min}$

12. $\dfrac{750 \text{ mL}}{4 \text{ hours}} \times \dfrac{10 \text{ gtts/mL}}{60 \text{ minutes}} = 31 \text{ gtts/min}$

13. $\dfrac{100 \text{ cc}}{45 \text{ minutes}} \times 20 \text{ gtts/mL} = 44 \text{ gtts/min}$

14. $\dfrac{50 \text{ mL}}{15 \text{ minutes}} \times 10 \text{ gtts/mL} = 33 \text{ gtts/min}$

15. $\dfrac{50 \text{ mL}}{1.5 \text{ hour}} \times \dfrac{60 \text{ gtts/mL}}{60 \text{ minutes}} = 33 \text{ gtts/min}$

16. $\dfrac{500 \text{ cc}}{3.5 \text{ hour}} \times \dfrac{10 \text{ gtts/mL}}{60 \text{ minutes}} = 23.8 \text{ or } 24 \text{ gtts/min}$

17. $\dfrac{20 \text{ mL}}{20 \text{ minutes}} \times 15 \text{ gtts/mL} = 15 \text{ gtts/min}$

18. $\dfrac{400 \text{ mL}}{6 \text{ hours}} \times \dfrac{60 \text{ gtts/mL}}{60 \text{ minutes}} = 67 \text{ gtts/min}$

19. $\dfrac{175 \text{ mL}}{90 \text{ minutes}} \times 20 \text{ gtts/mL} = 39 \text{ gtts/min}$

20. $\dfrac{150 \text{ cc}}{45 \text{ min}} \times 15 \text{ gtts/mL} = 49.9 \text{ or } 50 \text{ gtts/min}$

☐ More Practice Problems

1. Order: 1000 cc D$_5$W IV to run 8 hours.
   Administration set: 15 gtts/cc.

   For how many drops per minute should you regulate the IV?

2. Order: 1000 mL Normal Saline IV to run 6 hours.
   Administration set: 20 gtts/mL.

   For how many drops per minute should you regulate the IV?

3. Order: One pint of whole blood IV to run 4 hours.
   Equipment available: Blood Administration Set (10 gtts/cc).

   a. How many cc in a pint?

   b. How fast should the infusion be regulated to be completed in 4
      hours?

4. Order: #1 1000 cc D_5W
          #2 500 cc NS } IV
          #3 500 cc R/L

   Infuse the three IVs one after the other over 18 hours.
   Administration set: 15 gtts/cc.
   Calculate the drop rate so that the total amount is infused in the pre-
   scribed time.

5. Juanita is 2½ weeks old and is admitted to the hospital severely de-
   hydrated.
   Doctor's orders: 0.45% NaCl in 2.5% Dextrose in Water; 85 mL the
                    first hour; 200 mL q. 8. h. × 3 (less 85 mL ordered
                    the first hour).
   The infusion was started with a microdrop (60 gtts/mL).

   a. How fast must it run the first hour?

   b. How fast should it run for the remaining 7 hours?

c. How fast for the remaining two 8-hour periods?

6. Ordered: 1500 cc D$_5$ Plasmanate IV to run 10 hours.
   Administration set: 15 gtts/cc.

   For how many drops per minute must the IV be regulated to infuse at the appropriate rate?

7. An IV of 1000 cc Hartman's Solution is infusing at a rate of 125 cc/h. The administration set you use delivers 20 gtts/cc.

   What would be the gtts/min?

8. Order: 1000 cc N/S IV run at 90 cc/h.
   Available administration set: 10 gtts/cc.

   a. What is the correct drop rate?

   b. What would be the drop rate if you changed to a microdrop?

9. Order: 450 cc of D$_5$W IV over 3 hours.
   Administration set: 15 gtts/cc.

   What is the drop rate per minute?

10. The patient is to receive a transfusion of 3 units of packed cells. Each unit contains 250 cc. You begin the first unit at 9 am and by 1 pm the third unit should be infused.
    Special blood administration tubing set delivers 10 gtts/cc.

    What is the drop rate?

11. Order: 1000 cc D5W to alternate with 1000 cc D5RL over the next 24
    hours at a rate of 150 cc/h.
    Administration set: 20 gtts/cc.

    How many drops per minute?

12. Order: 1000 cc D_5R/L to run at 90 cc per hour.
    Administration set: 10 gtts/cc.

    At how many gtts/min should the IV run?

13. Order: 250 mg Aminophylline® (aminophylline) in 250 cc D_5W to run
    8 hours.
    Administration set: microdrop.

    At how many cc/h and drops per minute should the IV run?

14. Order: Keflin® (cephalothin sodium) 500 mg IV piggyback over one
    hour. Mix Keflin in 100 mL N/S.
    Equipment available: 15 gtts/mL.
    Note: The amount and/or type of solution used to mix the piggyback
    drug may not be included in the order. The nurse should consult the
    drug literature or the pharmacist to obtain the appropriate informa-
    tion.

    How fast should the Keflin drip?

15. Order: 1 Gm Keflin® (cephalothin sodium) in 50 mL of D_5W q.6.h.
    Equipment available: 20 gtts/mL.

    To infuse in 30 minutes, the nurse should regulate the infusion at what
    drop rate?

16. Order: 250 mg Achromycin® (tetracycline HCl) IV q. 12. hr.
    Dilute in 100 cc D5W and administer over a 30 minute period.
    Administration set available: 10 gtts/cc.

    How fast should the Achromycin infuse?

17. You have an order to give Rheomacrodex® (Dextran 40) 250 cc over 45 minutes.
    Administration set: 15 gtts/cc.

    What is the flow rate?

18. Order: Infuse Plasmanate® (plasma protein fraction) at a rate of 4 mL per min for a total of 500 mL.
    Administration set: 10 gtts/mL.

    What is the flow rate?

19. Order: Aminophylline® (aminophylline) 100 mg dissolved in 35 cc of NS to infuse in 45 minutes.
    Administration set: microdrop.

    What is the flow rate?

20. Order: Geopen® (carbenicillin disodium) 2 Gm IVPB. Dilute in 50 mL and administer over 15 minutes.
    Administration set: 20 gtts/mL.

    What is the flow rate?

21. Order: Pentam® (pentamidine isethionate) 250 mg in 100 mL of D5W IV once daily.
    Administration set: 15 gtts/mL.
    The literature states to give it over 60 minutes.

    For how many drops per minute should you regulate the IV?

22. Order: Mandol® (cefamandole nafate) in 100 mL of NS IV q6h over 30 minutes.
    Available administration set: 10 gtts/mL.

    For how many drops per minute should you regulate this IV?

23. Order: Tagamet® (cimetidine) 300 mg IVPB q.6.h.
    Mix in 50 mL D5W and infuse over 15 to 20 minutes.
    Administration set: 20 gtts/mL.

    What is the flow rate for:
    15 minutes

    20 minutes

24. Order: Administer 3 ampules of 5-mL ampules of Septra® (trimetho-
    prim & sulfamethoxazole) IV every 6 hours over 90 minutes.
    The literature states each 5 mL of Septra should be diluted in 125 mL
    of D5W.
    Administration set: 10 gtts/mL.

    a. How many mL of D5W will be needed to dilute the dosage?

    b. For how many drops per minute should you regulate the IV if you
       added the ampules to the above volume?

    c. If your patient was on strict fluid control and you must limit the
       total infusion to 375 mL, how much diluent would you require?

    d. What would be the flow rate for 375 mL?

    The literature states that for the disease for which this patient is re-
    ceiving this drug, the total daily dose is 15 to 20 mg/kg (based on the
    trimethoprim component) given in three or four equally divided doses.

Each 5-mL ampule contains 80 mg of trimethoprim and 400 mg of sulfamethoxazole.
Patient's weight: 50 kg.

e. Is this patient receiving a recommended dosage?

25. Order: Heparin Sodium Injection (heparin sodium) 40,000 U in 1000 mL of NS IV over 24 hours.
    Administration set: 60 gtts/mL.
    Available: Heparin Sodium Injection 10,000 units per mL.

    a. How many mL of Heparin Sodium will you add to the 1000 mL of IV solution?

    b. For how many drops per minute should you regulate the IV?

    c. How many units of Heparin is the patient receiving each hour?

26. Order: Garamycin® (gentamicin sulfate) 60 mg IVPB q 8 h.
    Available: Garamycin 80 mg per 2 mL.
    Administration set: 10 gtts/mL.

    a. How many mL of Garamycin will you prepare to equal the dosage ordered?

    b. You dilute the medication in NS to equal 150 mL. How many drops per minute to infuse in 1 hour?

27. Order: 2500 cc D5W over 12 hours.
    Administration set: 10 drops/mL.

    The IV was started at 0700, and 800 mL remain at 1500. To complete the IV within the scheduled time, how fast, in drops per minute, should the IV run?

☐ Answers

1. $\dfrac{1000 \text{ cc}}{8 \text{ hours}} \times \dfrac{15 \text{ gtts/cc}}{60 \text{ minutes}} = 31.2 \text{ or } 31 \text{ gtts/min}$

2. $\dfrac{1000 \text{ mL}}{6 \text{ hours}} \times \dfrac{20 \text{ gtts/ml}}{60 \text{ minutes}} = 55.5 = 56 \text{ gtts/min}$

3. a. 500 cc per pint

   b. $\dfrac{500 \text{ cc}}{4 \text{ hours}} \times \dfrac{10 \text{ gtts/cc}}{60 \text{ minutes}} = 20.8 \text{ or } 21 \text{ gtts/min}$

4. $1000 \text{ cc D}_5\text{W}$
   500 cc N/S
   $\underline{500 \text{ cc RL}}$
   2000 cc Total

   $\dfrac{2000 \text{ cc}}{18 \text{ hours}} \times \dfrac{15 \text{ gtts/cc}}{60 \text{ minutes}} = 27.7 \text{ or } 28 \text{ gtts/min}$

5. a. $\dfrac{85 \text{ mL}}{1 \text{ hour}} \times \dfrac{60 \text{ gtts/mL}}{60 \text{ minutes}} = 85 \text{ gtts/min*}$

   b. 200 mL/8 h
      $\underline{-85 \text{ mL first hour}}$
      $115 \text{ mL for 7 hours}$

      $\dfrac{115 \text{ mL}}{7 \text{ hours}} \times \dfrac{60 \text{ gtts/mL}}{60 \text{ minutes}} = 16.42 \text{ or } 16 \text{ gtts/min}$

   c. $\dfrac{200 \text{ mL}}{8 \text{ hours}} \times \dfrac{60 \text{ gtts/mL}}{60 \text{ minutes}} = $ 25 gtts/min for each of the remaining 8-hour periods

---

* Remember when using the microdrop, the cc or mL per hour equals the drops per minute.

6. $\dfrac{1500 \text{ cc}}{10 \text{ hours}} \times \dfrac{15 \text{ gtts/cc}}{60 \text{ minutes}} = 37.5 \text{ or } 38 \text{ gtts/min}$

7. $\dfrac{125 \text{ cc}}{1 \text{ hour}} \times \dfrac{20 \text{ gtts/cc}}{60 \text{ minutes}} = 41.6 \text{ gtts/min or } 42 \text{ gtts/min}$

8. a. $\dfrac{90 \text{ cc}}{1 \text{ hour}} \times \dfrac{10 \text{ gtts/cc}}{60 \text{ minutes}} = 15 \text{ gtts/min}$

   b. 90 gtts per minute. Remember the cc per hour equals the drops per minute with the microdrop.

9. $\dfrac{450 \text{ cc}}{3 \text{ hours}} \times \dfrac{15 \text{ gtts/cc}}{60 \text{ minutes}} = 37.5 \text{ or } 38 \text{ gtts/min}$

10. $\dfrac{750 \text{ cc}}{4 \text{ hours}} \times \dfrac{10 \text{ gtts/cc}}{60 \text{ minutes}} = 31.25 \text{ or } 31 \text{ gtts/min}$

11. $\dfrac{150 \text{ cc}}{60 \text{ minutes}} \times 20 \text{ gtts/cc} = 50 \text{ gtts/min}$

12. $\dfrac{90 \text{ cc}}{60 \text{ minutes}} \times 10 \text{ gtts/cc} = 15 \text{ gtts/min}$

13. $\dfrac{250 \text{ cc}}{8 \text{ hours}} = 31.25 \text{ cc/h, } 31 \text{ gtts/min}$

14. $\dfrac{100 \text{ mL}}{1 \text{ hour}} \times \dfrac{15 \text{ gtts/mL}}{60 \text{ minutes}} = 25 \text{ gtts/min}$

15. $\dfrac{50 \text{ mL}}{30 \text{ minutes}} \times 20 \text{ gtts/mL} = 33.3 \text{ or } 33 \text{ gtts/min}$

16. 100 cc: 30 minutes :: X cc : 1 minute

$$30 \text{ X} = 100$$

$$\text{X} = 3.3 \text{ cc/min}$$

   3.3 cc/min $\times$ 10 gtts/cc = 33 gtts/min

17. $\dfrac{250 \text{ cc}}{45 \text{ minutes}} \times 15 \text{ gtts/cc} = 83 \text{ gtts/min}$

18. $\dfrac{4 \text{ mL}}{1 \text{ minute}} \times 10 \text{ gtts/mL} = 40 \text{ gtts/min}$

19. $\dfrac{35 \text{ cc}}{45 \text{ minutes}} \times 60 \text{ gtt/min} = 46.6 \text{ or } 47 \text{ gtts/min}$

20. $\dfrac{50 \text{ mL}}{15 \text{ minutes}} \times 20 \text{ gtts/min} = 66.6 \text{ or } 67 \text{ gtts/min}$

21. $\dfrac{100 \text{ mL}}{60 \text{ minutes}} \times 15 \text{ gtts/mL} = 25 \text{ gtts/min}$

22. $\dfrac{100 \text{ mL}}{30 \text{ minutes}} \times 10 \text{ gtts/mL} = 33 \text{ gtts/min}$

23. 15 minutes

    $\dfrac{50 \text{ mL}}{15 \text{ minutes}} \times 20 \text{ gtts/mL} = 67 \text{ gtts/min}$

    20 minutes

    $\dfrac{50 \text{ mL}}{20 \text{ minutes}} \times 20 \text{ gtts/mL} = 50 \text{ gtts/min}$

    You could regulate the IV between 50 and 67 gtts/min.

24. a. 5 mL : 125 mL : : 15 mL (3 ampules) : X mL

    $$5 X = 1875$$
    $$X = 375 \text{ mL}$$

    b. 375 mL diluent + 15 mL drug = 390 mL total volume

    $\dfrac{390 \text{ mL}}{90 \text{ minutes}} \times 10 \text{ gtt/mL} = 43.3 \text{ or } 43 \text{ gtts/min}$

    c. 360 cc

    d. $\dfrac{375 \text{ mL}}{90 \text{ minutes}} \times 10 \text{ gtts/mL} = 41.6 \text{ or } 42 \text{ gtts/min}$

    e. 15 mg : 1 kg : : X mg : 50 kg

    $$1 X = 750 \text{ mg}$$

    OR

    20 mg : 1 kg : : X mg : 50 kg

    $$1 X = 1000 \text{ mg}$$

    Patient is receiving 4 doses of 240 mg each for a total of 960 mg per 24 hours. The patient is receiving a recommended dose.

25. a. 10,000 U : 1 mL : : 40,000 U : X mL

    $$10,000 X = 40,000$$
    $$X = 4 \text{ mL}$$

b. $\dfrac{1000 \text{ mL}}{24 \text{ hours}} \times \dfrac{60 \text{ gtts/mL}}{60 \text{ minutes}} = 41.6$ or 42 gtts/min

c. 40,000 U : 24 hours :: X U : 1 hour

$$24 \text{ X} = 40,000$$

$$\text{X} = 1666.6 \text{ U per hour}$$

26. a. 80 mg : 2 mL :: 60 mg : X mL

$$80 \text{ X} = 120$$

$$\text{X} = 1.5 \text{ mL}$$

b. $\dfrac{150 \text{ mL}}{1 \text{ hour}} \times \dfrac{10 \text{ gtts/mL}}{60 \text{ min}} = 25$ gtts/min

27. $\dfrac{800 \text{ cc}}{4 \text{ hours}} \times \dfrac{10 \text{ gtt/mL}}{60 \text{ min}} = \dfrac{8000}{240} = 33.3$ or 33 gtts/min

Administration by Concentration

Most continuous and intermittent infusions are ordered by milliliters per hour, but the order may specify a certain concentration of the drug per hour, per minute, or per mL (mg/h, unit/h, microgram per minute, or mg/mL). To administer the prescribed dosage, the nurse may have to reconstitute the drug and determine the volume of fluid needed for the appropriate concentration. Remember, you must translate the drug ordered in mg, Gm, or mcg into volume that can be dripped.

Example 1

Order: Levophed® (norepinephrine bitartrate) 2 μg/min.
Available: 500 cc D₅W with 2000 μg added.
Administration set: microdrop.
What is the drop rate?
The first step is to determine the number of cc in which the prescribed dose per minute is contained.

$$2000 \text{ μg} : 500 \text{ cc} :: 2 \text{ μg} : \text{X cc}$$

$$2000 \text{ X} = 1000$$

$$\text{X} = 0.5 \text{ cc}$$

You have determined that 2 μg is contained in 0.5 cc and is to be infused in one minute.
Next multiply the cc per minute (0.5 cc) by 60 gtt/cc (the microdrop rate).

$$0.5 \text{ cc per minute}$$
$$\times \quad 60 \text{ gtts/cc}$$

30 gtts per minute— the drop rate to
infuse the Levophed
at 2 μg per minute

Sometimes it is important for a drug to be prescribed according to the weight of the individual and then be administered at a specific concentration over time.

Example 2

Order: Zinacef® (cefuroxime) IV 75 mg/kg/day.
Administer: q 8 h over 30 minutes.
Available: Zinacef® 750 mg vial of powder. Dilute with 8 mL of sterile
water for an approximate concentration of 90 mg/mL and
add to 50-cc IV bag of D5W. Microdrop Administration Set.
Patient's weight: 110 lbs.

What is the infusion rate?

microdrops _____   electronic device _____

First convert lbs to kg:

2.2 lbs : 1 kg :: 110 lbs : X kg

2.2 X = 110

X = 50 kg

Next calculate the amount of drug per day:

75 mg × 50 kg = 3750 mg/day

The order is for q8h, so divide the total for the day 3750 mg by 3. This yields 1250 mg per dose.

Determine the total reconstituted volume (TRV):

90 mg : 1 mL :: 750 mg : X mL

90 X = 750

X = 8.3 mL TRV

Next determine the volume per dose:

750 mg : 8.3 mL :: 1250 mg : X mL

750 X = 10,375

X = 13.83 mL of the drug

Because the bottle has 750 mg, you will need to reconstitute two bottles, drawing 8.3 cc (750 mg) from one vial and 5.8 cc (500 mg) from the second.

Next add the Zinacef to the 50-mL IV bag for a total of 63.8 or 64 mL of IV fluid with medication. To calculate the rate:

$$\frac{64 \text{ mL (volume)}}{30 \text{ minutes}} \times 60 \text{ gtts/cc} = 128 \text{ gtts/min}$$

Note

mL/h and gtts/min are the same with microdrop. The displacement was very small for this problem and really would not have made a significant difference, but to be safe, always calculate the exact volume.

Example 3

Order: Staphcillin® (methicillin sodium) 320 mg IV q. 12. h. Administer over 20 minutes at the concentration of 20 mg/mL.

Available: A 1-Gm vial with the following directions for reconstitution: Add 1.5 mL Sterile Water for Injection to yield 2 mL. Buretrol IV infusion set.

a. How many cc of the available drug will you remove from the reconstituted vial to equal the dose? (Convert Gm to mg because drug was ordered in mg and it eliminates the possible error with decimals.)

$$1 \text{ Gm} = 1000 \text{ mg} : 2 \text{ mL} :: 320 \text{ mg} : X \text{ mL}$$

$$1000 \text{ X} = 640$$

$$X = 0.6 \text{ mL}$$

b. What is the total number of mL of fluid that should be administered over 20 minutes?

$$20 \text{ mg} : 1 \text{ mL} :: 320 \text{ mg} : X \text{ mL}$$

$$20 \text{ X} = 320$$

$$X = 16 \text{ mL total fluid to be infused}$$

c. How much diluent (IV fluid) should you add to the pure drug to equal the total volume?

$$\begin{array}{r} 16 \quad \text{mL total} \\ -0.6 \text{ (320 mg of drug)} \\ \hline 15.4 \text{ mL of fluid to add} \end{array}$$

d. How fast should you regulate the IV?

$$320 \text{ mg} : 20 \text{ minutes} :: X \text{ mg} : 1 \text{ minute}$$

$$20 \text{ X} = 320$$

$$X = 16 \text{ mg/min}$$

$$20 \text{ mg} : 60 \text{ gtts} :: 16 \text{ mg} : X \text{ gtts}$$

$$20 \text{ X} = 906$$

$$X = 48 \text{ gtts/min}$$

e. If you could use an electronic regulating device, what would be the mL/h?

$$16 \text{ mL} : 20 \text{ minutes} :: X \text{ mL} : 60 \text{ minutes}$$

$$20 \text{ X} = 960$$

$$X = 48 \text{ mL/h}$$

☐ Practice Problems

1. Order: Add 50 mEq of KCl (potassium chloride) to 100 cc of IV fluid and administer at a rate of 10 mEq per hour.
   Administration set: microdrop.

   What is the rate of flow in gtts/min?

2. Order: Kantrex® (kanamycin) IV 15 mg/kg/day in evenly divided doses q 12 h.
   Patient's weight: 25 kg.
   Available: Kantrex 333 mg/mL for parenteral administration.
   Administer by Soluset (60 gtts/mL) in 25 mL D5NS over 1 hour.

   How much Kantrex will you add to the Soluset for each dose? How fast would you set the IV?

3. Order: Cleocin® (clindamycin phosphate) 900 mg in 100 cc NS IVPB q 6 hr. Infuse at a rate of 10 mg/min.
   Administration set: 15 gtts/cc.

a. How many mL per minute will be infused?

b. For how many gtts/min will you regulate the IV?

4. Order: Aminophylline® (theophylline ethylenediamine) 500 mg in
      1000 mL of D5W. Infuse at 25 mg per hour.
   Available: Aminophylline 250 mg per 10 mL.

   a. How many mL of Aminophylline will you add to the 1000 mL of
      D5W?

   b. For how many drops per minute should you regulate the IV to
      infuse 25 mg of Aminophylline each hour?
      Administration set: 60 gtts/mL.

5. Order: Humulin R® (regular insulin) 5 units per hour IV.
   Administer at a rate of 25 mL per hour.
   Available: 500 cc NS and a vial of Humulin R insulin.

   a. How many units of insulin will you add to the NS?

   b. How fast would you set the IV?
      Administration set: 60 gtts/min.

6. Order: Chloromycetin® (chloramphenicol sodium succinate) 180 mg
      IV.
   Administer over 15 minutes at a concentration of 15 mg/cc.

Available: A 1-Gm/10 cc vial of Chloromycetin and Buretrol Administration Set. Dilute with 10 mL of Sterile Water for Injection.

a. How many cc of the available drug should you use?

b. What is the total number of cc of fluid to be administered over the
15 minutes?

c. How much diluent should you add to the drug in the Buretrol?

d. For how fast should you set the IV?

7. Order: Lidocaine® (lidocaine hydrochloride) 1 Gm in 250 cc D_5W IV.
The drug is to be administered at the rate of 2 mg/min.

Using a microdrop administration set, you should adjust the flow rate
at how many drops/min?

8. Order: Heparin Sodium (heparin sodium) 800 U per hour IV.
Available: Heparin Sodium 20,000 U in 500 cc D5W.
Administration set: microdrop.

a. How many cc per hour should you infuse?

b. For how many drops per minute should you regulate the IV?

9. Order: Diuril® (chlorothiazide sodium) 350 mg IV with 50 cc D5W. The Diuril is to be given at 15 mg/min.
   Administration set: 15 gtts/cc.

   How fast should the fluid drip?

10. Order: ACTH® (corticotropin injection) 15 units in 500 cc of Ringers Lactate.
    Administer at a rate of 0.06 U/min.
    Administration set: microdrop.

    a. How many cc should infuse in 1 minute?

    b. How many units per hour will be infused?

11. Order: Isuprel® (isoproterenol hydrochloride) 2 mcg/min.
    Available: Isuprel 2 mg per 250 ml NS.
    Administration set: microdrop.

    a. What is the rate in mL/min?

    b. What is the rate in mL/h?

12. Order: Humulin® R 50 Units in 500 mL NS. Infuse at 1 mL per minute.
    Administration set: 20 gtts/mL.

    a. What is the flow rate in gtts/min?

    b. How many units per hour is the patient receiving?

13. Order: Heparin sodium drip 40,000 U in 500 mL of 0.45% NS to infuse at 1200 U/h.
    Available: An electronic infusion device.

    What is the flow rate in mL/h?

14. Order: Pronestyl® (procainamide hydrochloride) 1 Gm in 500 mL D5W. Regulate at 4 mg/min.
    Available: An electronic infusion device.

    At how many mL/h should the medication infuse?

15. Order: Isuprel® (isoproterenol hydrochloride) 5 mcg/min IV.
    Available: Isuprel 2 mg in 500 mL D5W.

    What is the rate per hour?

16. Order: Lidocaine hydrochloride 1 g in 250 mL D5W. Regulate at 2 mg/min.
    Administration set: microdrop.

    How many drops per minute?

17. Order: Nitrostat® IV (nitroglycerin) 10 mcg/min IV.
    Available: Nitrostat IV 8 mg ampule, 250 mL of D5W and disposable IV infusion set with microdrop tubing.

    What would the drip rate be?

18. Order: Morphine sulfate 40 mg in 250 mL to infuse at 3 mg/h.
    Administration set: microdrop.

    How many drops per minute?

19. Order: Bretylol (bretylium tosylate) 5 mg/kg/body weight IV stat over
    45 minutes.
    Available: Bretylol 500 mg per 10-mL ampule.
    Patient's weight: 187 lbs.

    a. How many mg should this patient receive?

    b. How many mL of Bretylol will you prepare?

    c. For how many drops per minute should you regulate the IV? The
       literature says to dilute the contents or portion thereof in a min-
       imum of 50 mL D5W.
       Administration set: 60 gtts/mL.

20. Order: Tagamet® (cimetidine) 2 mg/kg/h IV. Add 2000 mg to
    1000 cc D5W.
    Administration set: 15 gtts/mL.
    Patient's weight: 140 lbs.

    a. How fast should you set the IV?

21. Order: Nipride® (nitroprusside sodium) 0.5 mcg/kg/min.
    Patient's weight: 125 lbs.

    a. How many mcg should the patient receive?

    The drug is added to fluid to equal a concentration of 100 mcg/mL.

    b. What is the rate in cc/h?

22. Intropin® (dopamine hydrochloride) is dripping at a rate of 25 cc/h.
    The concentration of Intropin is 200 mg in 250 mL.
    Patient's weight: 65 kg.

    What is the mcg/kg/min the patient is receiving?

23. Order: Dobutrex® (dobutamine) at 6 mcg/kg/min.
    Available: Dobutrex 250 mg in 250 cc D5W.
    Administration set: microdrop.
    Patient's weight: 50 kg.

    What is the drop rate in gtts/min _____ and cc/h _____ ?

24. Order: Intropin® (dopamine) 200 mg in 250 mL of NS. The patient is
    to receive 5 mcg/kg/min.
    Available: Microdrop and electronic flow regulator.
    Patient's weight: 132 lbs.

    a. At how many gtts per minute should the IV be regulated?

    b. At how many mL/hr would you set the electronic flow regulator?

25. Order: Aminophylline® (theophylline) 0.5 mg/kg/h IV.
    Available: Aminophylline 500 mg in 1000 cc D5W.
    Administration set: microdrop.
    Patient's weight: 70 kg.

    a. How many cc per hour should the patient receive?

    b. How many drops per minute?

26. Order: Humulin® R 100 U in 250 mL NS.
    Administer at 0.1 unit/kg/hr.
    Administration set: microdrop.
    Patient's weight: 110 lbs.

    a. How many units of Humulin R should the patient receive per hour?

    b. What is the drop rate?

27. Order: 350 mg Diuril® (chlorothiazide sodium) in 50 mL of D5W ad-
    ministered by Buretrol.
    Administer at 10 mg/min.
    Available: Diuril 0.5-Gm dry powder vial. Reconstitute with 18 mL
    Sterile Water for Injection.

    a. How many mL of the drug equal the dose?

    b. If the total amount of fluid to be infused is 50 mL, how much D5W
       should be added to the Buretrol?

    c. What would be the flow rate to administer 10 mg/min?

    d. If the ordered drug had been added to the 50 mL D5W, what would
       have been the drip rate?

☐ **Answers**

1. 50 mEq : 100 cc : : 10 mEq : X cc

$$50 X = 1000$$

$$X = 20 \text{ cc/h}$$

$$\frac{20 \text{ cc/h}}{60 \text{ min}} \times 60 \text{ gtts/min} = 20 \text{ gtts/min}$$

2. 25 kg × 15 mg = 375 mg/day ÷ 2 (q 12 hours) = 187.5 mg/dose

333 mg : 1 mL : : 187.5 mg : X mL

$$333 X = 187.5$$

$$X = 0.56 \text{ mL of the pure drug}$$

$$\frac{25 \text{ mL}}{1 \text{ hour}} \times \frac{60 \text{ gtt/mL}}{60 \text{ minutes}} = 25 \text{ gtts/min}$$

3. a. 900 mg : 100 cc : : 10 mg : X cc

$$900 X = 1000$$

$$X = 1.1 \text{ cc/min}$$

   b. 15 gtts : 1 mL : : X gtts : 1.1 cc

$$1 X = 16.5 \text{ or } 17 \text{ gtts/min}$$

4. a. 250 mg : 10 mL : : 500 mg : X mL

$$250 X = 5000$$

$$X = 20 \text{ mL}$$

   b. 500 mg : 1000 mL : : 25 mg : X mL

$$500 X = 25,000$$

$$X = 50 \text{ mL}$$

$$\frac{50 \text{ mL}}{1 \text{ hour}} \times \frac{60 \text{ gtts/mL}}{60 \text{ minutes}} = 50 \text{ gtts/min}$$

5. a. 5 U : 25 mL : : X U : 500 mL

$$25 X = 2500$$

$$X = 100 \text{ units added to the IV}$$

   b. $\dfrac{25 \text{ mL}}{1 \text{ hour}} \times \dfrac{60 \text{ gtts/mL}}{60 \text{ minutes}} = 25 \text{ gtts/min}$

6. a. 1000 mg : 10 cc :: 180 mg : X cc

$$1000 \text{ X} = 1800$$

$$\text{X} = 1.8 \text{ cc}$$

b. 15 mg : 1 cc :: 180 mg : X cc

$$15 \text{ X} = 180$$

$$\text{X} = 12 \text{ cc total}$$

c. $\begin{array}{r} 12 \quad \text{cc total volume} \\ -\,1.8 \text{ cc of drug} \\ \hline 10.2 \text{ cc of diluent} \end{array}$

d. 180 mg : 15 minutes :: X mg : 1 minute

$$15 \text{ X} = 180$$

$$\text{X} = 12 \text{ mg/min}$$

OR

(cc/h) 12 cc : 15 minutes :: X cc : 60 minutes

$$15 \text{ X} = 720$$

$$\text{X} = 48 \text{ cc/h}$$

15 mg : 60 gtts :: 12 mg : X gtts

$$15 \text{ X} = 720$$

$$\text{X} = 48 \text{ gtts/min}$$

OR

(gtt/min) 48 cc/h ÷ 60 minutes = $\begin{array}{r} 0.8 \text{ cc/min} \\ \times\ 60 \text{ gtts/mL} \\ \hline 48.0 \text{ gtts/min} \end{array}$

7. 1000 mg : 250 cc :: 2 mg : X cc

$$1000 \text{ X} = 500$$

$$\text{X} = 0.5 \text{ cc per minute}$$

60 gtts : 1 cc :: X gtts : 0.5 cc

$$\text{X} = 30 \text{ gtts/min}$$

8. a. 20,000 U : 500 cc :: 800 U : X cc

$$20,000 \text{ X} = 400,000$$

$$\text{X} = 20 \text{ cc per hour}$$

b. $\dfrac{20 \text{ cc}}{60 \text{ min}} \times 60 \text{ gtts/cc} = 20 \text{ gtts/min}$

9. 350 mg : 50 cc : : 15 mg : X cc

$$350 \text{ X} = 750$$

$$\text{X} = 2.14 \text{ cc/min}$$

2.14 cc/min $\times$ 15 gtts/cc = 32.1 or 32 gtts/min

10. a. 15 U : 500 cc : : 0.06 U : X cc

$$15 \text{ X} = 30$$

$$\text{X} = 2 \text{ cc}$$

b. 0.06 U : 1 minute : : X U : 60 minutes

$$1 \text{ X} = 3.6 \text{ U/h}$$

11. a. 1000 mcg : 1 mg : : X mcg : 2 mg

$$1 \text{ X} = 2000 \text{ mcg}$$

2000 mcg : 250 mL : : 2 mcg : X mL

$$2000 \text{ X} = 500$$

$$\text{X} = 0.25 \text{ mL}$$

b. 0.25 cc/min $\times$ 60 minutes = 15 cc/h

12. a. 1 mL/min $\times$ 20 gtts/mL = 20 gtts/min

b. 1 mL/min $\times$ 60 min/h = 60 mL/h

50 units : 500 mL : : X units : 60 mL

$$500 \text{ X} = 3000$$

$$\text{X} = 6 \text{ units per hour}$$

13. 40,000 U : 500 mL : : 1200 U : X mL

$$40,000 \text{ X} = 600,000$$

$$\text{X} = 15 \text{ mL/h}$$

14. 1 Gm = 1000 mg : 500 mL : : 4 mg : X mL

$$1000 \text{ X} = 2000$$

$$\text{X} = 2 \text{ mL/min} \times 60 \text{ min} = 120 \text{ mL/h}$$

15. 2 mg = 2000 mcg : 500 mL :: 5 mcg : X mL

$$2000 \text{ X} = 2500$$

$$\text{X} = 1.25 \text{ mL/min}$$

5 mcg = 1.25 ml × 60 min/h = 75 mL/h

16. 1000 mg : 250 mL :: 2 mg : X mL

$$1000 \text{ X} = 500$$

$$\text{X} = 0.5 \text{ mL}$$

0.5 mL : X gtts :: 1 mL : 60 gtts/mL

$$\text{X} = 30 \text{ gtts/min}$$

17. 8 mg = 8000 mcg : 250 mL :: 10 mcg : X mL

$$8000 \text{ X} = 2500$$

$$\text{X} = 0.3125 \text{ mL} \times 60 \text{ gtts/mL}$$

$$= 18.75 \text{ or } 19 \text{ gtts/min}$$

18. 40 mg: 250 mL :: 3 mg : X mL

$$40 \text{ X} = 750$$

X = 18.75 mL = 19 cc/h (with a microdrop, the cc/h are equal to drops/min, 19 gtts/min)

19. 187 lbs = 85 kg

 a. 5 mg : 1 kg :: X mg : 85 kg

$$1 \text{ X} = 425 \text{ mg}$$

 b. 500 mg : 10 mL :: 425 mg : X mL

$$500 \text{ X} = 4250$$

$$\text{X} = 8.5 \text{ mL}$$

 c. 50 mL D5W + 8.5 mL of the drug = 58.5 total volume

$$\frac{58.5 \text{ mL}}{45 \text{ minutes}} \times 60 = 78 \text{ mL/h or } 78 \text{ gtts/min}$$

If you add the entire ampule (10 mL) to the 50 mL D5W and then calculate the dosage, you would get the following results.

50 mL D5W + 10 mL of drug = 60 mL total

500 mg : 60 mL : : 425 mg : X mL

500 X = 25,500

X = 51 cc to be infused
(total volume of medication
and IV fluid = 60 mL)

To prevent administering too much medication, you must subtract 9 cc from the IV container and then regulate the IV.

$$\frac{51 \text{ cc}}{45 \text{ minutes}} \times 60 \text{ gtts/mL} = 67.9 \text{ or } 68 \text{ gtts/min}$$

20. a. 140 lbs = 63.6 kg

63.6 kg × 2 mg = 127.2 mg/h

2000 mg : 1000 cc : : 127.2 mg : X cc

2000 X = 127,200

X = 63.6 or 64 cc/h

$$\frac{64 \text{ cc}}{60 \text{ minutes}} \times 15 \text{ gtts/mL} = 15.9 \text{ or } 16 \text{ gtts/min}$$

21. a. 125 lbs = 56.8 kg
56.8 kg × 0.5 mcg = 28.4 mcg/min

b. 100 mcg : 1 mL : : 28.4 mcg : X mL

100 X = 28.4

X = 0.284 mcg/mL × 60 min = 17.04 cc/h

22. a. 200 mg = 200,000 mcg

200,000 mcg : 250 mL : : X mcg : 25 cc

250 X = 5,000,000

X = 20,000 mcg/h

20,000 mcg : 60 minutes : : X mcg : 1 minute

60 X = 20,000

X = 333.33 mcg/min

333.33 mcg/min/65 kg = 5.13 mcg/kg/min

23. 250,000 mcg : 250 cc :: 6 mcg : X cc

$$250,000 \; X = 1500$$

$$X = 0.006 \; cc$$

0.006 cc × 50 kg = 0.3 cc/min × 60 gtts/mL = 18 gtts/min

0.3 cc/min × 60 min/h = 18 cc/h

24. 132 lbs = 60 kg   5 mcg × 60 kg = 300 mcg/min

   a. 200 mg = 200,000 mcg : 250 mL :: 300 mcg : X mL

$$200,000 \; X = 75000$$

$$X = 0.375 \; mL/min$$

  0.375 mL × 60 gtt/mL = 22.5 or 23 gtts/min

   b.   0.375 mL = 5 mcg/kg/min

       × 60 min/h

     22.5 or 23 mL/h

25. a. 0.5 mg × 70 kg = 35 mg/h

   500 mg : 1000 cc :: 35 mg : X cc

$$500 \; X = 35,000$$

$$X = 70 \; cc/h$$

  b. $\dfrac{70 \; cc}{1 \; hour} \times \dfrac{60 \; gtt/mL}{60 \; minutes} = 70 \; gtts/min$

26. a. 50 kg × 0.1 units = 5 units/h

  b. 100 U : 250 mL :: 5 U : X mL

$$100 \; X = 1250$$

$$X = 12.5 \; mL/h$$

  12.5 mL : 60 minutes :: X mL : 1 minute

$$60 \; X = 12.5$$

$$X = 0.208 \; mL/min \times 60 \; gtts$$

$$= 12.49 \; or \; 12.5 \; or \; 13 \; gtts/min$$

27. a. 500 mg (0.5 g) : 18 mL :: 350 mg : X mL

$$500 \; X = 6300$$

$$X = 12.6 \; mL$$

b.   50   mL total volume
   $\underline{- 12.6 \text{ Diuril in solution}}$
   37.4 mL D5W

c. 350 mg : 50 mL :: 10 mg : X mL

$$350 \text{ X} = 500$$

$$\text{X} = 1.4 \text{ mL/min} \times 60 \text{ gtts}$$

$$= 84 \text{ gtts/min}$$

d.   50   mL D5W
   $\underline{+ 12.6 \text{ mL Diuril in solution}}$
   62.6 total volume

350 mg : 62.6 mL :: 10 mg : X mL

$$350 \text{ X} = 626$$

$$\text{X} = 1.78 \text{ or } 1.8 \text{ mL/min} \times 60 \text{ gtts}$$

$$= 108 \text{ gtts/min}$$

Other Intravenous Calculations

Intravenous infusions are regulated and monitored carefully to ensure that the fluids and medications are delivered in a specific time period. Many factors may cause the infusion to be ahead of or behind schedule. When you find that the infusion is not on schedule, you will be expected to follow your agency procedure on readjusting the flow rate. In most cases, if the increase or decrease in rate does not exceed 25% of the original rate, the nurse may recalculate the flow rate to complete the infusion within the originally ordered time period.

Type 1

At report the nurse stated that she hung 1000 cc D5W at 1430 at a rate of 125 cc/h. At 1530 the IV was infusing on time. Checking the infusion at 1730, the nurse found 700 cc remained. At 125 cc/h approximately 375 cc should have been infused and 625 cc should remain to infuse.
Administration set: 20 gtts/cc.

a. How long should the original IV have run?

$$\frac{1000 \text{ cc}}{125 \text{ cc/h}} = 8 \text{ hours}$$

b. Recalculate the IV to complete on time.

The IV should have been completed at 2230 hours. At this time 5 hours remain of the original 8 hours.

$$\frac{700 \text{ cc}}{5 \text{ hours}} \times \frac{20 \text{ gtts/cc}}{60 \text{ min/h}} = 46.6 \text{ or } 47 \text{ gtts/min}$$

Sometimes the nurse may need to determine:

- How long the IV will infuse at the current rate.

- How much medication the patient is receiving per hour or minute at the current rate.

Type 2

IV of D5W is infusing at 35 gtts/min, 600 cc remain in the bottle. Administration set: 10 gtts/mL.

At this rate, how long will it take to infuse? _____ hours _____ minutes

First convert the drops into cc:

$$35 \text{ gtts} : X \text{ cc} :: 10 \text{ gtts} : 1 \text{ cc}$$
$$10 \text{ X} = 35$$
$$X = 3.5 \text{ cc/min}$$
$$3.5 \text{ cc} : 1 \text{ minute} :: 600 \text{ cc} : X \text{ minutes}$$
$$3.5 \text{ X} = 600$$
$$X = 171.4 \text{ or } 171 \text{ minutes}$$
$$60 \text{ minutes} : 1 \text{ hour} :: 171 \text{ minutes} : X \text{ hours}$$
$$60 \text{ X} = 171$$
$$X = 2.85 \text{ hours (2 hours and 0.85}$$
$$\text{or } 0.9 \text{ hour)}$$
$$\text{(Multiply } 0.9 \text{ hour by } 60 \text{ min/h} = 54 \text{ minutes.)}$$
$$= 2 \text{ hours and } 54 \text{ minutes}$$

If you are comfortable with the formula method for determining drop rate, you can put the information into the formula and solve for X. *You must remember the rules for solving for X.*

Using the same information from previous problem.

$$\frac{600 \text{ cc (volume)}}{X \text{ hours}} \times \frac{10 \text{ gtts/mL (drop factor)}}{60 \text{ min/h}} = 35 \text{ gtts/min}$$

$$X = \frac{600 \text{ cc} \times 10 \text{ gtts}}{35 \text{ gtts} \times 60 \text{ minutes}} = \frac{6000}{2100} = 2.857 \text{ or } 2.9$$

2 hours and .9 × 60 minutes = 2 hours and 54 minutes

Type 3

The electronic flow regulator is set at 30 mL/h.
Available: Dopastat® (dopamine hydrochloride) 400 mg in 500 mL NS.
Patient's weight: 165 lbs.

How many mcg/kg/min is the patient receiving?

Convert lbs to kg:

$$2.2 \text{ lbs} : 1 \text{ kg} :: 165 \text{ lbs} : X \text{ kg}$$

$$2.2 X = 165$$

$$X = 75 \text{ kg}$$

Solve for mcg/mL:

Find out how many mcg/mL are available:

1000 mcg = 1 mg

$$400,000 \text{ mcg} : 500 \text{ mL} :: X \text{ mcg} : 1 \text{ mL}$$

$$500 X = 400,000$$

$$X = 800 \text{ mcg/mL}$$

Solve for mcg/kg:

$$800 \text{ mcg} : 75 \text{ kg} :: X \text{ mcg} : 1 \text{ kg}$$

$$75 X = 800$$

$$X = 10.7 \text{ mcg/kg}$$

Solve for mcg/kg/min:

$$10.7 \text{ mcg} : 1 \text{ mL} :: X \text{ mcg} : 30 \text{ mL}$$

$$1 X = 321 \text{ mcg/h}$$

$$321 \text{ mcg} : 60 \text{ min} :: X \text{ mcg} : 1 \text{ min}$$

$$60 X = 321$$

$$X = 5.35 \text{ mcg/kg/min}$$

☐ **Practice for Type 1 Problems**

For each of the situations below, determine the amount of time each IV should run if continued at the current drop rate.

	Current Drop Rate (gtts/min)	Administration Set (gtts/mL)	Fluid Remaining (mL)	Time (hours and minutes)
1.	30	10	500	
2.	25	15	750	
3.	27	20	600	
4.	12	15	450	
5.	33	10	500	
6.	20	60	80	
7.	36	20	350	
8.	32—	10	650	

	Current Drop Rate (gtts/min)	Administration Set (gtts/mL)	Fluid Remaining (mL)	Time (hours and minutes)
9.	50	10	1000	
10.	20	15	250	

☐ Answers

1. 30 gtts : X mL :: 10 gtts : 1 mL

$$10 X = 30 \quad X = 3 \text{ mL per minute}$$

3 mL : 1 minute :: 500 mL : X minutes

$$3 X = 500 \quad X = 166.6 \text{ or } 167 \text{ minutes}$$

60 minutes : 1 hour :: 167 minutes : X hours

$$60 X = 167$$

$$X = 2.78 \text{ or } 2.8 \text{ hours } (0.8 \times 60 \text{ min} = 48 \text{ min})$$
$$= 2 \text{ hours and } 48 \text{ minutes}$$

2. $\dfrac{750 \text{ mL}}{X \text{ hours}} \times \dfrac{15 \text{ gtts/mL}}{60 \text{ minutes}} = 25 \text{ gtts/min}$

$$X = \frac{750 \text{ mL} \times 15 \text{ gtts/mL}}{25 \text{ gtts/min} \times 60 \text{ minutes}}$$

$$= 7.5 \text{ hours } (0.5 \times 60 = 30 \text{ min})$$
$$= 7 \text{ hours } 30 \text{ minutes}$$

3. 27 gtts: X mL :: 20 gtts : 1 mL

$$20 X = 27, \quad X = 1.35 \text{ mL/min}$$

1.35 mL : 1 minute :: 600 mL : X minutes

$$1.35 X = 600$$

$$X = 444.4 \text{ minutes} \div 60$$
$$= 7.4 \text{ hours } (0.4 \times 60 = 24 \text{ min})$$
$$= 7 \text{ hours } 24 \text{ minutes}$$

4. $\dfrac{450 \text{ mL}}{\text{X hours}} \times \dfrac{15 \text{ gtts/mL}}{60 \text{ min/h}} = 12 \text{ gtts/min}$

$X = \dfrac{450 \times 15}{12 \times 60} = \dfrac{6750}{720} = 9.375 \text{ or } 9.4 \text{ hours}$

$(0.4h \times 60 \text{ min/h} = 24 \text{ min})$

$= 9 \text{ hours and } 24 \text{ minutes}$

5. 10 gtts : 1 mL : : 33 gtts : X mL

$10 \text{ X} = 33$

$X = 3.3 \text{ mL/min}$

3.3 mL : 1 minute : : 500 cc : X minutes

$3.3 \text{ X} = 500$

$X = 151.5 \text{ or } 152 \text{ minutes} \div 60 \text{ min/h}$

$= 2.53 \text{ or } 2.5 \text{ hours or } 2 \text{ hours } 30 \text{ minutes}$

6. $\dfrac{80 \text{ mL}}{\text{X hours}} \times \dfrac{60 \text{ gtts/mL}}{60 \text{ min/h}} = 20 \text{ gtts/min}$

$X = \dfrac{80 \times 60}{20 \times 60} = 4 \text{ hours}$

7. 20 gtts : 1 mL : : 26 gtts : X mL

$20 \text{ X} = 26$

$X = 1.3 \text{ mL/min}$

1.3 mL : 1 minute : : 350 mL : X minutes

$1.3 \text{ X} = 350$

$X = 269.23 \text{ or } 269 \text{ minutes} \div 60 \text{ min/h}$

$= 4.48 \text{ or } 4.5 \text{ hours or } 4 \text{ hours and } 30 \text{ minutes}$

8. $\dfrac{650 \text{ mL}}{\text{X hours}} \times \dfrac{10 \text{ gtts/mL}}{60 \text{ min/h}} = 32 \text{ gtts/min}$

$X = \dfrac{650 \times 10}{32 \times 60} = \dfrac{6500}{1920} = 3.385 \text{ hours}$

$= 3.4 \text{ hours } (0.4h \times 60 \text{ min/h} = 24 \text{ min})$

$= 3 \text{ hours and } 24 \text{ minutes}$

9. 10 gtts : 1 mL : : 50 gtts : X mL

$10 \text{ X} = 50$

$X = 5 \text{ mL/min}$

5 mL : 1 minute : : 1000 mL : X minutes

$$5\,X = 1000$$

$$X = 200 \text{ minutes} \div 60 \text{ min/h}$$

$$= 3.33 \text{ hours} = 3 \text{ hours and } 20 \text{ minutes}$$

10. $\dfrac{250 \text{ mL}}{\text{X hours}} \times \dfrac{15 \text{ gtts/mL}}{60 \text{ min/h}} = 20 \text{ gtts/min}$

$X = \dfrac{250 \times 15}{20 \times 60} = \dfrac{3750}{1200} = 3.125 \text{ or } 3 \text{ hours and } 8 \text{ minutes}$

The exact minutes may vary slightly depending how many decimals you use. We recommend always using two decimals and then rounding at the end of the problem. You should round off to whole minutes.

If you missed more than two of these problems go back and review. You should determine which method (proportion or formula) of solving the problems is the easiest for you and stick to that method.

☐ Practice for Type 2 and 3 Problems

1. Mrs. Jones' IV of 1000 cc R/L was started at 8 a.m. to run for 12 hours. It is now 3 p.m. and 800 cc remain in the bottle.

   a. In order to infuse the IV in the 12 hours, how fast would it have to drip if you had equipment that delivered 15 gtts/cc?

   b. How much fluid should have been infused by this time?

   c. If you were to calculate the infusion rate for the fluid that remained at 3 p.m. keeping within the original 12-hour schedule, how fast would you have to set the IV?

2. 750 mL remain in an IV, which is dripping at 21 gtts/min. The IV equipment being used is 10 gtts/mL. At this rate, how many hours will it take to complete the infusion?

3. The physician ordered 500 cc of a special electrolyte solution to flow at 50 gtts/min. The pharmacy has called to ask how long before you will need the next bottle.
   Administration set: 15 gtts/cc.

   How long will it take to infuse the 500 cc?

4. You check the IV and 450 cc remain. The IV is dripping at 18 gtts/min and the administration set is calibrated to deliver 15 gtts/mL.

   At the present rate, how long will it take the IV to infuse?

5. Heparin® (heparin sodium) is running at 25 gtts/min.
   Available: Heparin 30,000 U in 500 ml D5W.
   Administration set: microdrop.

   How many units of Heparin is the patient receiving per hour?

6. Order: 1000 cc D5RL was started at 1500 hours.
   Administration set: 15 gtts/cc.
   At 1800 hours, 350 cc remain, and it is dripping at 44 gtts/min.

   At this rate, what time will the IV be completed?

7. The controller is set at 38 mL/h.
   Available: Dopastat® (dopamine hydrochloride) 400 mg in 500 mL NS.
   Patient's weight: 198 lbs.

   How many mcg/kg/min is the patient receiving?

8. The electronic flow regulator is set at 25 cc/h.
   Available: Nipride® (nitroprusside) 50 mg in 250 cc D5W.
   Patient's weight: 132 lbs.

   How many mcg/kg/min is the patient receiving?

9. The IV is dripping at 15 gtts/min.
   Available: Dobutrex® (dobutamine) 250 mg in 250 cc D5W.
   Patient's weight: 70 kg.

   How many mcg/kg/min is the patient receiving?

10. The IV is infusing at 40 gtts/min.
    Available: 250 cc D5W with 200 mg of Intropin® (dopamine).
    Administration set: microdrop.
    Patient's weight: 165 lbs.

    At this rate, how many mcg/kg/min will the patient receive?

☐ **Answers**

1. a. $\dfrac{1000 \text{ cc}}{12 \text{ hours}} \times \dfrac{15 \text{ gtts/cc}}{60 \text{ minutes}} = 20.8 \text{ or } 21 \text{ gtts/min}$

   b. 83 cc/h or 581 cc

   c. $\dfrac{800 \text{ cc}}{5 \text{ hours}} \times \dfrac{15 \text{ gtts/cc}}{60 \text{ minutes}} = 40 \text{ gtts/min}$

2. 21 gtts ÷ 10 gtts/mL = 2.1 cc/min

   750 cc ÷ 2.1 cc = 357 minutes or 5.9 or 6 hours

3. 50 gtts: X cc :: 15 gtts : 1 cc

    15 X = 50

    X = 3.3 cc per minute

    3.3 cc : 1 minute :: X cc : 60 minutes

    X = 198 cc/h

    198 cc : 1 hour :: 500 cc : X hours

    198 X = 500

    X = 2.52 or 2 hours 30 minutes

4. 18 gtts : X mL :: 15 gtts : 1 mL

$$15 X = 18$$

$$X = 1.2 \text{ mL/min}$$

1.2 mL/min $\times$ 60 min/h = 72 cc/h

450 cc $\div$ 72 cc/h = 6 hours and 15 minutes

5. 30,000 units : 500 cc :: X units : 1 cc

$$500 X = 30,000$$

$$X = 60 \text{ units/cc}$$

60 units : 60 gtts (1 cc) :: X units : 25 gtts

$$60 X = 1500$$

$$X = 25 \text{ units/min} \times 60 = 1500 \text{ units/h}$$

6. $\dfrac{350 \text{ mL}}{X \text{ time}} \times \dfrac{15 \text{ gtts/mL}}{60 \text{ minutes}} = 44 \text{ gtts/min}$

$$X = \frac{350 \times 15}{44 \times 60} = \frac{5250}{2640}$$

$$= 1.98 \text{ or 2 hours or at 2000 hours}$$

7. 198 lbs = 90 kg

400,000 mcg (400 mg) : 500 mL :: X mcg : 1 mL

$$500 X = 400,000$$

$$X = 800 \text{ mcg/mL}$$

800 mcg : 90 kg :: X mcg : 1 kg

$$90 X = 800$$

$$X = 8.8 = 9 \text{ mcg/kg}$$

9 mcg : 1 mL :: X mcg : 38 mL

$$X = 342 \text{ mcg/h} \div 60 \text{ min/h} = 5.7 \text{ mcg/min}$$

8. 132 lbs = 60 kg

50,000 mcg (50 mg) : 250 cc :: X mcg : 1 cc

$$250 X = 50,000$$

$$X = 200 \text{ mcg/cc}$$

200 mcg : 60 kg : : X mcg : 1 kg

$$60 \text{ X} = 200$$

$$\text{X} = 3.3 \text{ mcg/kg}$$

3.3 mcg : 1 cc : : X mcg : 25 cc

$$\text{X} = 82.5 \text{ mcg/h} \div 60 \text{ minutes} = 1.375 \text{ or } 1.4 \text{ mcg/min}$$

9. 250,000 mcg (250 mg) : 250 cc: : X mcg : 1 cc

$$250 \text{ X} = 250,000$$

$$\text{X} = 1000 \text{ mcg/cc}$$

1000 mcg : 70 kg : : X mcg : 1 kg

$$70 \text{ X} = 1000$$

$$\text{X} = 14.28 \text{ or } 14.3 \text{ mcg/kg}$$

14.3 mcg : 60 gtts : : X mcg : 15 gtts

$$60 \text{ X} = 214.5$$

$$\text{X} = 3.575 \text{ or } 3.6 \text{ mcg/kg/min}$$

10. 165 lbs = 75 kg

200,000 mcg (200 mg) : 250 mL : : X mcg : 1 mL

$$250 \text{ X} = 200,000$$

$$\text{X} = 800 \text{ mcg/mL}$$

800 mcg : 75 kg : : X mcg : 1 kg

$$75 \text{ X} = 800$$

$$\text{X} = 10.6 \text{ mcg/kg}$$

10.6 mcg : 60 gtts : : X mcg : 40 gtts

$$60 \text{ X} = 424$$

$$\text{X} = 7.1 \text{ mcg/kg/min}$$

Administration of Medications by IV Push

A drug given IV push in a peripheral vein reaches the heart and is pumped to the brain in approximately 15 minutes. The patient receives almost immediate benefit from the drug. The physician's order for IV push medication rarely contains the infusion time. The infusion time is usually determined by the nurse, who is guided by agency policy and/or current pharmacology literature. Most IV push medications should be administered over a period of 1 to 5 minutes (maybe longer) but NEVER less than 1 minute. The volume of the prescribed drug should be calculated to increments of 15- to 30-second intervals so the nurse can use a watch that displays seconds or with a second hand to provide a smooth and accurate administration.

The actual skill of administering IV push medications is beyond the scope of this text. For specific techniques used to administer medications IV push consult the hospital procedure manual or an advanced clinical skills textbook.

Example 8

Order: Tagamet® (cimetidine) 300 mg IV push now.
Available: Tagamet 300 mg/2 mL.
The literature recommends diluting the Tagamet to a total of 20 mL. Compatible solution recommended: Sodium Chloride Injection (0.9%). Inject over a period of not less than 2 minutes. An injection time of 5 minutes was selected.

a. How many mL of Tagamet equal 300 mg?

$$2 \text{ mL}$$

b. How many mL of Sodium Chloride must you add to equal desired volume?

$$\begin{array}{r} 20 \text{ mL desired} \\ -\ 2 \text{ mL dosage} \\ \hline 18 \text{ mL amount to add} \end{array}$$

Check the literature carefully to determine if the volume of the drug is in addition to the diluent or a part of the total diluent. For example, the total volume of diluent + drug is 20 mL in this problem. If the literature states to dilute in 20 mL then the total volume would be 22 mL (drug + diluent).

c. To complete the infusion in 5 minutes how many mL should you infuse every minute?

$$20 \text{ mL} : 5 \text{ minutes} :: X \text{ mL} : 1 \text{ minute}$$

$$5 X = 20$$

$$X = 4 \text{ mL per minute}$$

d. To ensure a smooth and accurate administration how much should you infuse every 15 seconds?

$$4 \text{ mL} : 60 \text{ seconds} :: X \text{ mL} : 15 \text{ seconds}$$
$$60 \text{ X} = 60$$
$$X = 1 \text{ cc every 15 seconds}$$

☐ Practice Problems

1. Order: Coumadin® (warfarin sodium) 0.75 mg/kg IV push STAT.
   Patient's weight: 70 kg.
   Available: Coumadin 50-mg powder per vial. Dilute each 50 mg with
       2 mL.
   Rate of administration: 25 mg or fraction thereof over 1 minute.

   a. How many mg should the patient receive?

   b. How many mL should you administer?

   c. How many mL per minute should you infuse?

   d. How many mL should you infuse each 15 seconds?

2. Order: Amytal Sodium® (amobarbital sodium) 750 mg IV push NOW.
   Each 125 mg must be diluted with 1.25 mL of Sterile Water for Injection.
   Recommended rate of administration: Each 100 mg or fraction of a mg
   administer over 1 minute.

   a. What is the total volume you should administer?

   b. You should administer the drug over _____ minutes.

   c. How many mL should you administer?
     Every minute ____; every 30 seconds ____; every 15 seconds ____

3. Order: Aquamephyton® (phytonadione) 5 mg IV push now.
   Available: Aquamephyton 10 mg/mL.
   The literature states the drug should be diluted in at least 10 mL of NS and administered at a rate of 1 mg or fraction thereof per minute.

   a. How much diluent should you add to the medication?

   b. How many mL of Aquamephyton equals the prescribed dose?

   c. How much medication should you inject every 30 seconds to infuse the drug at 1 mg/min?

4. Order: Digoxin 0.375 mg IV push at a rate of 1 mL/min.
   Available: Digoxin ampule of 0.25 mg/mL.
   Directions: Dilute each mL in 4 mL of sterile water.

   a. How many mL of Digoxin would you administer?

   b. How much time would it take to administer the Digoxin?

5. Order: Valium® (diazepam) 20 mg IV titrated at 5 mg/min.
   Available: Valium 5 mg/mL ampule.

   a. How much time would it take to infuse the dose?

   b. How much would you administer every 15 seconds?

☐ **Answers**

1. a. 0.75 mg : 1 kg :: X mg : 70 kg

    X = 52.5 mg

   b. 50 mg : 2 mL :: 52.5 mg : X mL

    50 X = 105

    X = 2.1 mL

   c. 2.1 mL/3 minutes = 0.7 mL/minute

   Remember the 0.1 is a fraction, so the total time should be 3 minutes.

   d. 0.7 mL : 60 seconds :: X mL : 15 seconds

    60 X = 10.5

    X = 0.175 or 0.2 mL per 15 seconds

2. a. 125 mg : 1.25 mL :: 750 mg : X mL

    125 X = 937.5

    X = 7.5 cc total volume

   b. 100 mg : 1 minute :: 750 mg : X minutes

    100 X = 750

    X = 7.5 = 8 minutes

   c. 7.5 mL : 8 minutes :: X mL : 1 minute

    8 X = 7.5

    X = 0.9 mL per minute

   0.9 ÷ 2 = 0.45 mL per 30 seconds

   0.9 ÷ 4 = 0.225 mL per 15 seconds

3. a. 10 mL diluent

   b. 10 mg : 1 mL :: 5 mg : X mL

    10 X = 5

    1 X = 0.5 mL Aquamephyton

   c. 1 mg : 60 seconds :: X mg : 30 seconds

    60 X = 30

    X = 0.5 mL/30 seconds

4. a. 0.25 mg : 1 mL :: 0.375 mg : X mL

   0.25 X = 0.375

   X = 1.48 or 1.5 mL of the drug

   b. 4 mL of diluent : 1 mL :: X mL diluent : 1.5 mL

   X = 6 mL of diluent

   6 mL diluent + 1.5 mL drug = 7.5 mL

   Administer at 1 mL per minute or over 7.5 minutes or 0.25 mL per 15 seconds.

5. a. 5 mg : 1 minute :: 20 mg : X minutes

   5 X = 20

   X = 4 minutes

   b. 1 mL : 60 seconds :: X mL : 15 seconds

   60 X = 15

   X = 0.25 mL per 15 seconds

Calculating Dosages for Infants and Children

Infants and children require smaller quantities of drugs than adults. Although the physician prescribes the specific drug and dose to be given, it is the responsibility of the nurse to recognize incorrect dosages and to contact the physician.

A combination of age in years or months, an average adult weight (150 lbs), and the average adult dose of the drug was the basis for calculating the appropriate drug dosage for infants and children for many years. This method did not always elicit the most therapeutic dose for a child, because the child, due to illness, might not follow the average developmental schedule for age. Also, the term "little adult" is not appropriate when referring to the physiology of infants and children. Research has led manufacturers to calculate doses for infants and children by a more exact method, body weight in kilograms and/or body surface area. The average adult dose still remains a factor when research has not established a specific pediatric dose.

Determining Pediatric Dose by Weight

If you are responsible for administering medications to infants and children, it is important to have an accurate current weight. Remember that the patient should be weighed on the same scale with the same amount of clothing and preferably at the same time daily. The scales may weigh in pounds (lb) or kilograms (kg). Drugs are commonly ordered in milligrams, micrograms, or M^2 (body surface area) per kilogram of body weight in evenly divided doses over a 24-hour period. To calculate the correct dosage the weight in pounds must be converted to kilograms.

Remember: 2.2 pounds = 1 kilogram. To change pounds to kilograms, divide the pounds by 2.2.

Example: Child's weight: 35 pounds. What is her weight in kilograms?

$$2.2 \text{ lbs} : 1 \text{ kg} :: 35 \text{ lbs} : X \text{ kg}$$

$$2.2 X = 35$$

$$X = 15.90909 = 15.91 \text{ kg}^*$$

Since drug manufacturers recommend therapeutic dosage by weight and the physician may not have an accurate weight, the medication order may be stated:

Demerol 1.5 mg/kg IM on call to OR

For hospitals using a unit dose system, the order will be interpreted and filled by the pharmacy. Although the pharmacy may have requested the weight of the patient and dispensed a prefilled syringe, it is still the responsibility of the nurse who administers the drug to double-check and make sure that the amount dispensed is the correct dose not only in mg/kg but in volume.

In addition to calculation and verification of single doses, the nurse must be aware of the amount of the drug being received over a 24-hour period. It is important that the drug be given according to the recommended divided doses (eg, 0.5 mg/kg/day in 4 evenly divided doses would be interpreted to mean the total amount of the drug divided by 4 and that amount given every 6 hours). By determining the overall dose and the individual dose, the nurse is also verifying if the drug ordered is less than or greater than the recommended dose. When there is a difference (less than or greater than) in the ordered and the recommended dose, the nurse should consult the physician.

Example 1

The recommended dose of Demerol (meperidine) for an IM preop is 1.5 mg/kg.

How many mg should a child weighing 8 pounds receive?

a. Convert pounds to kilograms:

$$2.2 \text{ lbs} : 1 \text{ kg} :: 8 \text{ lbs} : X \text{ kg}$$

$$2.2 X = 8$$

$$X = 3.636, X = 3.64 \text{ kg}$$

b. Calculate recommended dose:

$$1.5 \text{ mg} : 1 \text{ kg} :: X \text{ mg} : 3.64 \text{ kg}$$

$$X = 5.46 \text{ mg}$$

---

* It is recommended to always carry out the decimal to at least 3 places and then round to 2 decimal places. This small difference in weight could be very important with some drugs administered to children.

How many mL should you administer?

Available: Demerol 25 mg/mL; 50 mg/mL; 75 mg/mL; 100 mg/mL.
Which drug concentration should you choose?

25 mg/mL

Note

Remember that you should select the concentration that will give you a volume appropriate for the patient and measurable volume. A child of 8 lbs does not have a great deal of muscle mass and a small volume is recommended.

Amount to administer:

$$25 \text{ mg} : 1 \text{ mL} :: 5.46 \text{ mg} : X \text{ mL}$$

$$25 X = 5.46$$

$$X = 0.218 = 0.22 \text{ mL}$$

To be accurate in your measurement, always use a tuberculin syringe for volume under 1 mL.

Look at the two syringes shown in Figure 11.1 to see why the TB syringe would provide the most accurate measure.

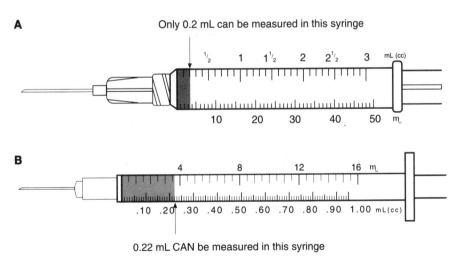

A Only 0.2 mL can be measured in this syringe

B

0.22 mL CAN be measured in this syringe

FIGURE 11.1.

Example 2

The recommended dose of children's Tylenol Elixir® (acetaminophen) is 10 mg/kg/dose. Each 5 mL contains 160 mg of the drug. How many mL would you administer to a child weighing 9 lbs 8 oz?

a. Convert pounds to kilograms. First change the ounces to percent of a pound:

$$16 \text{ oz} : 1 \text{ lb} :: 8 \text{ oz} : X \text{ lb}$$

$$16 X = 8$$

$$X = 0.5 \text{ lb}$$

$$2.2 \text{ lbs} : 1 \text{ kg} :: 9.5 \text{ lbs} : X \text{ kg}$$

$$2.2 X = 9.5$$

$$X = 4.32 \text{ kg}$$

b. Calculate recommended dose:

$$10 \text{ mg} : 1 \text{ kg} :: X \text{ mg} : 4.32 \text{ kg}$$

$$X = 43.2 \text{ mg}$$

c. Calculate amount of drug to give:

$$5 \text{ mL} : 160 \text{ mg} :: X \text{ mL} : 43.2 \text{ mg}$$

$$160 X = 216$$

$$X = 1.35 \text{ or } 1.4 \text{ mL Tylenol}$$

Because this is such a small volume, it should be measured on one of the specially designed calibrated spoons or droppers. Figure 11.2 shows how the above order should be measured.

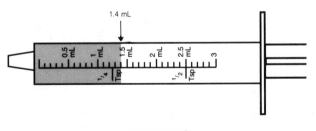

FIGURE 11.2.

With many drugs, the manufacturer will not provide an exact dose per kilogram but give you a range that is considered safe and therapeutic. In this situation, the nurse should calculate the minimum and maximum dose recommended and then compare that information to the order. A note of caution: Be sure to compare the single dose and the total recommended dose per day.

Example 3

Jane weighs 36 pounds. She has recently had surgery and has an order for 4 mg Morphine® (morphine sulfate) IM q4h PRN for pain. The product information indicates that a safe dose is 0.05 to 0.2 mg/kg.

What is the minimum dose?
First convert lbs to kg:

$$2.2 \text{ lbs} : 1 \text{ kg} :: 36 \text{ lbs} : X \text{ kg}$$

$$2.2 \text{ X} = 36$$

$$X = 16.36 \text{ kg}$$

Minimum dose:

$$16.36 \text{ kg} \times 0.05 \text{ mg} = 0.8 \text{ mg}$$

Maximum dose:

$$16.36 \text{ kg} \times 0.2 \text{ mg} = 3.27 \text{ mg}$$

Is the dose ordered (4 mg) within the safe range?
   NO, the maximum is 3.27 mg; the nurse should consult with the physician.

Example 4

Order: Pro-Banthine® (propantheline) 15 mg po q6h.
Available: Pro-Banthine 7.5- and 15-mg tablets.
Child's weight: 18 kg.
Recommended Dose: 1–2 mg/kg/day in four divided doses

How many mg are ordered for the day?
At every 6 hours (4 divided doses) the child will receive 60 mg per day.

What is the recommended dose per day?
   Minimum:

$$1 \text{ mg} : 1 \text{ kg} :: X \text{ mg} : 18 \text{ kg (child's weight)}$$

$$X = 18 \text{ mg per day}$$

Divided into 4 doses = 4.5 mg per dose

Maximum:

$$2 \text{ mg} : 1 \text{ kg} :: X \text{ mg} : 18 \text{ kg}$$

$$X = 36 \text{ mg per day}$$

Divided into 4 doses = 9 mg per dose

What is the difference in the ordered and the recommended dose?

	Dose	*Total Per Day*
Ordered:	15 mg	60 mg
Recommended:	4.5–9 mg	18–36 mg

The ordered amount is almost double the recommended dose and should be clarified with the physician before it is given. The medication comes in two strengths, 7.5 and 15 mg per tablet. If the prescribed dose was 7.5 mg q6h, this would equal 30 mg/day. This would fall within the therapeutic range of 18 mg to 36 mg per day and does not exceed the single-dose limit or 4.5 to 9 mg.

As you can see, when verifying the order, the nurse must check the dose carefully and also the amount to be administered.

☐ Practice Problems

1. Order: Demerol® (meperidine hydrochloride) 1 mg/kg IM STAT.
   Child's weight: 33 pounds.
   Available drug: Demerol 25 mg/mL.

   How many mL of Demerol should you administer?

2. Order: Tegretol® (carbamazepine) 200 mg po BID.
   The manufacturer recommends 30 mg/kg/day in two doses.
   Available in chewable-scored 100 mg tablets.
   Child's weight: 25 kg.

   Is the dose prescribed reasonable for the child?

3. Valium® (diazapam) 3.75 mg was ordered for a child with status epilipticus. The recommended dose is 0.2–0.5 mg/kg IV, slowly every 2–5 minutes, up to a maximum of 5 mg.
   Child's weight: 33 pounds.
   Available drug: Valium 5 mg/mL.

   a. How many mL should you administer to equal the ordered dose?

   b. Is the ordered dose within the therapeutic range?

4. Order: Septra Suspension® (trimethoprim and sulfamethoxazole) 20 ml po q12h.
   The literature states that each 5 mL of Septra Suspension contains 40 mg of trimethoprim and 200 mg of sulfamethoxazole. The usual dose for a child is 8 mg/kg of trimethoprim and 40 mg/kg of sulfamethoxazole per 24 hours given in two divided doses q 12h.
   Child's weight: 66 pounds.

   a. What is the recommended dose for trimethoprim?

   b. What is the ordered dose for trimethoprim?

   c. What is the recommended dose for sulfamethoxazole?

   d. What is the ordered dose for sulfamethoxazole?

   e. Is the dosage ordered above, below, or at the recommended amount?

5. Order: Luminal® (phenobarbital) 100 mg po q12h.
   The manufacturer recommends a maintenance dose of 3–5 mg/kg/day.
   The child weighs 30 kg.

   Is the prescribed dose within the therapeutic range?

6. The physician ordered Dilantin® (phenytoin) 4–8 mg/kg/day divided into two doses.
   An infant weighed 7 lb 2 oz.
   Available: Dilantin Suspension 30 mg/5 mL.

a. How many kg does the infant weigh?

b. What is the RANGE of the recommended dose per day?

c. How many mL should you administer for the maximum dose?

d. Indicate on the device shown in Figure 11.3 the amount from part c.

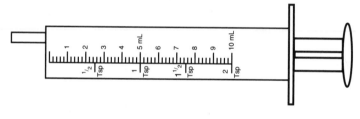

FIGURE 11.3.

7. Order: Ceclor® (cefaclor) 200 mg po q8h.
   Available: Ceclor 375 mg/5 mL suspension.
   Child's weight: 15 kg.
   Manufacturer information recommends a total daily dose of 20 to 40 mg per kg, in divided doses q 8–12h (maximum dose 1 g/day).

   a. What is the recommended LOWEST dose?

   b. How many mg should be administered per dose?

   c. What is the recommended HIGHEST dose?

d. How many mg should be administered per dose?

e. According to the order what is the total dose in milligrams the patient should receive each day?

f. Is the prescribed dose within the therapeutic range?

☐ **Answers**

1. 33 lbs = 15 kg

$$1 \text{ mg} \times 15 \text{ kg} = 15 \text{ mg Demerol}$$
$$25 \text{ mg} : 1 \text{ mL} :: 15 \text{ mg} : X \text{ mL}$$
$$25 X = 15$$
$$X = 0.6 \text{ mL}$$

2. Recommended dose:

$$30 \text{ mg} \times 25 \text{ kg} = 750 \text{ mg per day or } 375 \text{ mg per dose (BID)}$$

Ordered dose:

$$200 \text{ mg} \times 2 \text{ doses} = 400 \text{ mg per day}$$

The dose ordered is less than recommended and should be discussed with the physician.

3. 33 lbs = 15 kg

a. $5 \text{ mg} : 1 \text{ mL} :: 3.75 \text{ mg} : X \text{ mL}$

$$5 X = 3.75$$
$$X = 0.75 \text{ mL}$$

b. $15 \text{ kg} \times 0.2 \text{ mg} = 3 \text{ mg minimum dose range}$

$15 \text{ kg} \times 0.5 \text{ mg} = 7.5 \text{ mg maximum dose range}$

The ordered amount is within the acceptable range.

4. 66 lbs = 30 kg

   a. Trimethoprim
     Recommended:

$$8 \text{ mg} : 1 \text{ kg} :: X \text{ mg} : 30 \text{ kg}$$

$$X = 240 \text{ mg trimethoprim/24 hours}$$

   b. Ordered:

$$5 \text{ mL} : 40 \text{ mg} :: 20 \text{ mL} : X \text{ mg}$$

$$5 X = 800$$

$$X = 160 \text{ mg of trimethoprim q 12 hours}$$
$$\text{for a total of 320 mg/24 hours}$$

   c. Sulfamethoxazole
     Recommended:

$$40 \text{ mg} : 1 \text{ kg} :: X \text{ mg} : 30 \text{ kg}$$

$$X = 1200 \text{ mg of sulfamethoxazole/24 hours}$$

   d. Ordered:

$$5 \text{ mL} : 200 \text{ mg} :: 20 \text{ mL} : X \text{ mg}$$

$$5 X = 4000$$

$$X = 800 \text{ mg of sulfamethoxazole q 12 hours}$$
$$\text{for a total of 1600 mg/24 hours}$$

   e. The patient is receiving ABOVE the recommended amount of the drug.

5. Recommended:
   3 mg/kg/day

$$3 \text{ mg} \times 30 \text{ kg} = 90 \text{ mg/kg/day}$$

5 mg/kg/day

$$5 \text{ mg} \times 30 \text{ kg} = 150 \text{ mg/kg/day}$$

Ordered:

$$100 \text{ mg} \times 2 \text{ (q12h)} = 200 \text{ mg/day}$$

The ordered dose is greater than the recommended dose.

6. a. Convert oz to percent of pound:

$$2 \text{ oz} : X \text{ lb} :: 16 \text{ oz} : 1 \text{ lb}$$

$$16 X = 2$$

$$X = 0.125 \text{ or } 0.13 \text{ pounds}$$

Change pounds to kilograms:

$$9.13 \text{ lbs} : X \text{ kg} :: 2.2 \text{ lbs} : 1 \text{ kg}$$

$$2.2 \text{ X} = 9.13$$

$$X = 4.15 \text{ kg}$$

b. Recommended:
4 mg/kg/day

$$4 \text{ mg} \times 4.15 \text{ kg} = 16.6 \text{ mg}$$

8 mg/kg/day

$$8 \text{ mg} \times 4.15 \text{ kg} = 33.2 \text{ mg}$$

c. Maximum dose:

$$30 \text{ mg} : 5 \text{ mL} :: 33.2 \text{ mg} : X \text{ mL}$$

$$30 \text{ X} = 166$$

$$X = 5.53 \text{ mL}$$

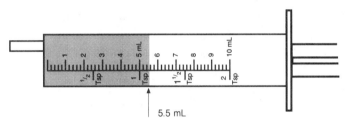

5.5 mL

FIGURE 11.4.

7. a. Lowest dose:

$$20 \text{ mg} : 1 \text{ kg} :: X \text{ mg} : 15 \text{ kg}$$

$$X = 300 \text{ mg total daily dose}$$

b. 300 mg/3 doses = 100 mg per dose

c. Highest dose:

$$40 \text{ mg} : 1 \text{ kg} :: X \text{ mg} : 15 \text{ kg}$$

$$X = 600 \text{ mg total daily dose}$$

d. 600 mg/3 doses = 200 mg per dose

e. Total dose per day:

$$200 \text{ mg} \times 3 \text{ (q8h)} = 600 \text{ mg total daily dose}$$

f. Yes, 600 mg is at the maximum of the therapeutic range.

Body Surface Area

The Body Surface Area (BSA) formula may be used to calculate therapeutic drug dosages for adults or children. Each child and each drug should be considered individually. Sometimes children require the same dose of a drug as an adult, but in most cases the dosage is reduced. BSA is commonly used with chemotherapeutic drugs.

In the absence of nomograms, charts, or tables to determine Body Surface Area, the following formula may be used:

$$\frac{\text{(Four time child's weight in kilograms)} + 7}{\text{(Children's weight in kilograms)} + 90} = \frac{\text{Body Surface Area}}{\text{in square meters (m}^2)}$$

Note

In the drug company literature m^2 is used when they are determining the dose according to the BSA (Body Surface Area).

Example 1

Determine the Body Surface Area of a child weighing 30 lbs.
30 lbs = 13.6 kg

$$\frac{(4 \times 13.6) + 7}{13.6 + 90} = \frac{54.4 + 7}{13.6 + 90} = \frac{61.4}{103.6} = 000.59 \text{ BSA in m}^2$$

Note

1. Remember, in working with fractions you must add and subtract before you multiply and divide.
2. To divide fractions you invert and multiply.

Example 2

The usual adult dose of Phenobarbital (phenobarbital) is gr iss po TID.
Available: Phenobarbital Elixir 20 mg/5 mL.
Child's weight: 48 lbs.

What is the recommended dose according to Body Surface Area?
48 lbs = 21.8 kg

$$\frac{(4 \times 21.8) + 7}{21.8 + 90} = \frac{87.2 + 7}{111.8} = \frac{94.20}{111.8} = 0.84 \text{ BSA (m}^2)$$

Once the Body Surface Area has been determined, the following formula should be used to determine the child's dose:

$$\frac{\text{Surface area in square meters}}{1.7^*} \times \frac{\text{Usual}}{\text{adult dose}} = \frac{\text{Child's}}{\text{dose}}$$

$$\frac{0.84 \text{ BSA}}{1.7} \times 100 \text{ mg}(1\frac{1}{2} \text{ gr}) = 49.4 \text{ mg TID}$$

Once the correct dose for the child has been determined, use the proportion formula to calculate the specific amount of the drug to equal each dose.

How many mL should you administer per dose?

$$20 \text{ mg} : 5 \text{ mL} :: 49.4 \text{ mg} : X \text{ mL}$$

$$20 X = 247$$

$$X = 12.35 \text{ or } 12.4 \text{ mL}$$

☐ Practice Problems

8. The usual adult dose of Dilantin® (phenytoin sodium) is 300 mg/day. Available: Dilantin-125 suspension 125 mg/5 mL.

   a. How much should be ordered for a child weighing 75 lbs?

   b. How many mL should you administer per dose if given t.i.d.?

9. The usual IM adult dose of Unipen® (nafcillin sodium) is 500 mg q6h.

   a. How many Gm per 24 hours?

   b. What is the BSA for a child weighing 88 lbs?

---

* 1.7 is the average BSA of an adult.

c. What would be the correct dose for the child for a 24-hour period?

d. How many mg should the child receive q.4.h.?

10. The usual adult maintenance dose of Crystodigin® (digitoxin) is 0.15 mg po daily.
    Available: Crystodigin 0.05-mg and 0.1-mg scored tablets.
    Child's weight: 13 kg.

    a. What is the Body Surface Area (m²)?

    b. How much should a child weighing 13 kg receive per dose?

11. The usual adult dose of Kefzol® (cefazolin sodium) is 500 mg q 6–8 hours.
    Available: Kefzol labeled as shown in Figure 11.5.

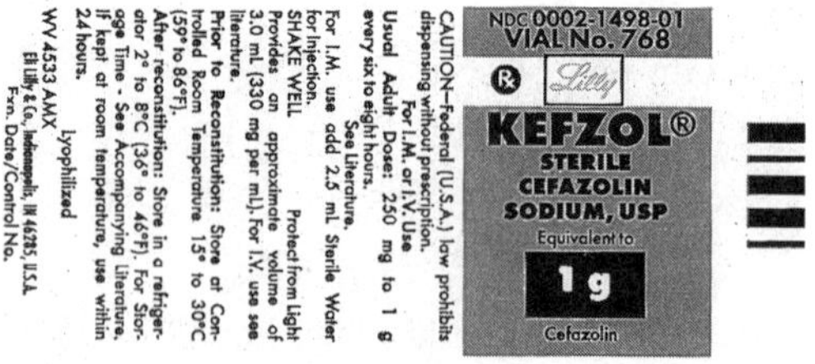

FIGURE 11.5.

Child's weight: 33 lbs.

a. What is the BSA (m²)?

b. How many mL should you administer per dose to a child weighing 33 pounds?

c. What syringe would allow for the most precise measurement?

12. The recommended dose of Calcijex® (calcitriol injection) for IV use in children is 0.05 mcg/kg/day until discontinued.
Available: Calcijex labeled as shown in Figure 11.6.

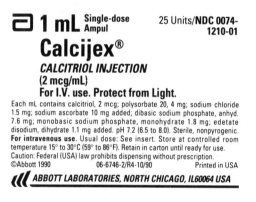

FIGURE 11.6.

How many mL should a child who weights 55 lbs receive each day?

13. The following is a typical preoperative medication for an adult:

Demerol® (meperidine hydrochloride) 100 mg $\Big\}$ IM on call
Thorazine® (chlorpromazine) 25 mg

The drugs are available in the following strengths:

Demerol 50 mg/mL
Thorazine 25 mg/mL

Child's weight: 25 lbs.

a. How many milligrams would you give of Demerol and Thorazine?

b. How many minims of these drugs would you administer?

c. What would be total volume of the mixed drugs?

14. Order: Cleocin® (clindamycin phosphate) 75 mg IM q6h.
    Available: Cleocin 150 mg/mL.
    The manufacturer recommends giving 350 mg/m^2/day to a maximum of 450 mg/m^2/day for a child.
    Child's weight: 13.6 kg.

    a. How many mg of the drug are ordered over 24 hours?

    b. What is the recommended dose range?

    c. Is the prescribed dose reasonable?

15. The usual adult dose of Ilotycin® (erythromycin) is 2 Gm/day (dose range from 1–4 Gm/day).
    Available: Ilotycin 250-mg tablets (unscored).

    a. What is the recommended dose for a child weighing 32 kg?

    b. Given the recommended dose of medication and the available tablets, how much would you give each dose if the order read to administer BID?

16. The doctor has ordered 10 mg Morphine® (morphine sulfate) for a child who weighs 19 kg. The adult dose is 8–20 mg. Is the prescribed dose within the safe range for the child?

☐ **Answers**

8. 75 lb = 34.1 kg

$$\frac{(4 \times 34.1) + 7}{34.1 + 90} = \frac{143.4}{124.1} = 1.16 \text{ BSA}$$

a. $\dfrac{1.16}{1.7} \times 300$ mg = 204.7 or 205 mg/day or 68 mg/dose

b. 125 mg : 5 mL :: 68 mg : X mL

$$125 \text{ X} = 340$$

$$\text{X} = 2.7 \text{ mL per dose}$$

9. 88 lbs = 40 kg

a. 6 Gm

b. $\dfrac{(4 \times 40) + 7}{40 + 90} = \dfrac{167}{130} = 1.28 \text{ BSA}$

c. $\dfrac{1.28}{1.7} \times 6$ Gm = 4.5 Gm/24 hours

d. Approximately 750 mg q.4.h.

10. a. $\dfrac{(4 \times 13) + 7}{13 + 90} = \dfrac{52 + 7}{103} = \dfrac{59}{103} = 0.573 \text{ BSA}$

b. Patient should receive one 0.05-mg tablet daily

$$\frac{0.57 \text{ BSA}}{1.7} \times 0.15 = 0.05 \text{ mg}$$

11. 33 pounds = 15 kilograms

a. $\dfrac{(4 \times 15) + 7}{15 + 90} = \dfrac{60 + 7}{105} = \dfrac{67}{105} = 0.638$ BSA

b. $\dfrac{0.638 \text{ BSA}}{1.7} \times 500 \text{ mg} = 187.5$ mg per dose

330 mg : 1 mL :: 187.5 mg : X mL

330 X = 187.5

X = 0.568 or 0.57 mL

c. Tuberculin syringe measures in hundredths

12. 55 lbs = 25 kg
0.05 mcg × 25 kg = 1.25 mcg/day
Available is Calcijex 2 mcg/mL

2 mcg : 1 mL :: 1.25 mcg : X mL

2 X = 1.25

X = 0.625 or 0.63 mL

13. 25 lbs = 11.36 kg

$$\dfrac{(4 \times 11.36) + 7}{11.36 + 90} = \dfrac{52.44}{101.36} = 0.517 \text{ BSA}$$

a. Demerol

$$\dfrac{0.517 \text{ BSA}}{1.7} \times 100 \text{ mg} = 30.4 \text{ mg of drug}$$

Thorazine

$$\dfrac{0.517 \text{ BSA}}{1.7} \times 25 \text{ mg} = 7.6 \text{ mg of drug}$$

b. Demerol

50 mg : 16 ℳ :: 30.4 mg : X ℳ

50 X = 486.4

X = 9.728 or 9.7 = 10 minims

Thorazine

25 mg : 16 ℳ :: 7.6 mg : X ℳ

25 X = 121.6

X = 4.86 or 5 minims

c. 10 ℳ Demerol

<u> 5 ℳ Thorazine </u>

15 ℳ Total Volume

14. $\dfrac{(4 \times 13.6) + 7}{13.6 + 90} = \dfrac{61.4}{103.6} = 0.59$ BSA

    a. 75 mg × 4 doses (q6h) = 300 mg per 24 hours

    b. Recommended dose:

$$350 \text{ mg} \times 0.59 \text{ BSA} = 206.5 \text{ mg per day}/4$$
$$= 51.6 \text{ mg or } 52 \text{ mg per dose}$$

Maximum dose:

450 mg × 0.59 BSA = 265.5 mg per day/4 = 66 mg per dose

    c. The prescribed dose EXCEEDS the recommended dose.

15. $\dfrac{(4 \times 32) + 7}{32 + 90} = \dfrac{128 + 7}{122} = \dfrac{135}{122} = 1.106$ BSA

    a. $\dfrac{1.106 \text{ BSA}}{1.7} \times 2000 \text{ mg (2 Gm)} = 1301.1 \text{ or } 1301 \text{ mg/day}$

    b. 1301 mg/2 (BID) = 650.5 or 651 mg per dose

        250 mg : 1 tab :: 651 mg : X tab

              250 X = 651

                X = 2.6 tablets

The tablets are unscored; you can give two 250 mg tablets q12h for a total of 1000 mg (1 Gm)/day. This would be within the therapeutic range. To be more exact, you could give 2 tablets at one dose and 3 tablets at the next dose, but consult the physician.

16. BSA

$$\dfrac{(4 \times 19) + 7}{19 + 90} = \dfrac{83}{109} = 0.76 \text{ BSA}$$

8 mg

$$\dfrac{0.76 \text{ BSA}}{1.7} \times 8 \text{ mg} = 3.57 \text{ or } 3.6 \text{ mg}$$

20 mg

$$\dfrac{0.76 \text{ BSA}}{1.7} \times 20 \text{ mg} = 8.94 \text{ mg}$$

The dose of 10 mg exceeds the safe range of 3.6 mg to 8.9 mg.

Nomogram to Calculate Body Surface Area

The easiest way to determine a child's Body Surface Area (BSA) is to use a nomogram, such as the West Nomogram. To use the nomogram certain information must be available: height in inches or centimeters and weight in pounds or kilograms.

To determine the Body Surface Area of the patient:
1. Find the height (inches or centimeters) in the left-hand column.

2. Find the weight (pounds or kilograms) in the right-hand column.

3. Place a ruler between the height on the left and the weight on the right.

4. Draw a line from point to point.

5. Read the point where the line crosses the surface area (SA) scale. Count the increments very carefully. The surface area is reported in M^2 (square meters).

Look at the nomogram shown in Figure 11.7 and review the steps in determining the Body Surface Area for the following examples.

Example 1

Child's height: 40″.
Child's weight: 15 kilograms.
m^2: 0.66.

Example 2

Child's height: 70 cm.
Child's weight: 10 lbs.
m^2: 0.3.

Example 3

Child's height: 190 cm.
Child's weight: 70 kilograms.
m^2: 1.95.

If the child is of normal height for weight, you can use the inner scale on the Nomogram. Find the weight of the child in pounds and draw a line straight across to determine the Body Surface Area m^2.

Example 4

Child's height: normal for weight.
Child's weight: 27 lbs.
m^2: 0.54.

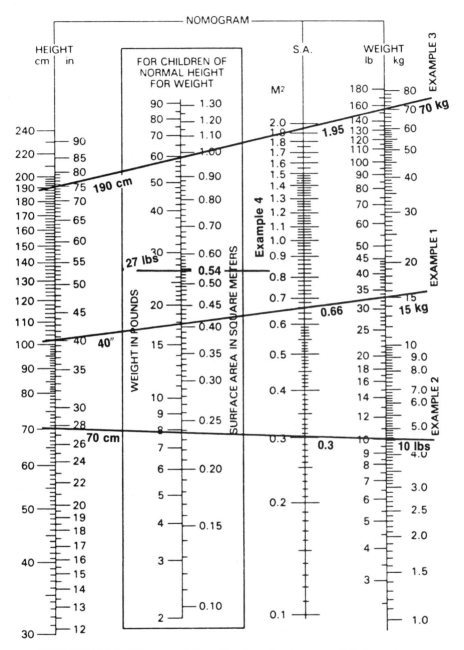

FIGURE 11.7. West Nomogram (for estimation of surface areas). Surface area is indicated where a straight line connecting height and weight intersects surface area (S.A.) column, or if patient is approximately of normal proportion, from weight alone (enclosed area). *(Nomogram modified from data of E. Boyd by C.D. West; from Behrman RE (ed): Nelson Textbook of Pediatrics, 14th ed. Philadelphia: Saunders, 1992, p. 1827.)*

Once the body surface area has been determined, the following formula should be used to determine the child's dose:

$$\frac{\text{Surface area in square meters}}{1.7^*} \times \text{Usual adult dose} = \text{Child's dose}$$

Example

a. Calculate the dose of a drug for a child weighing 30 lbs.
   The usual adult dose is 2 Gm.
   BSA = 0.59

$$\frac{0.59}{1.7} \times 2 \text{ Gm} = 0.694 \text{ Gm or 694 mg.}$$

Drug available in 1 Gm/2.2 mL:

$$1 \text{ Gm} : 2.2 \text{ mL} :: 0.69 \text{ Gm} : X \text{ mL}$$

$$X = 1.52 \text{ or } 1.5 \text{ mL}$$

b. Calculate the dose of a drug for a child with a body surface area of 1.20. The usual adult dose is 500 mg q. 12. hr (1 Gm/24 hours).

$$\frac{1.20}{1.7} \times 1 \text{ Gm} = 0.7058 \text{ Gm or 706 mg/24 hours or 353 mg q.12.h}$$

Drug available in 500 mg/mL:

$$500 \text{ mg} : 1 \text{ mL} :: 353 \text{ mg} : X \text{ mL}$$

$$500 X = 353$$

$$X = 0.7 \text{ mL}$$

Once the correct dose for the child has been determined, use the proportion formula to calculate the specific amount of the drug to equal each dose.

☐ Practice Problems

Use the Nomogram (Fig. 11.8) to determine BSA and solve the following problems.

17. Child's height: 45 inches.
    Child's weight: 42 pounds.
    Adult dose: 15 mg of drug.

    BSA:

    Child's dose:

---

* 1.7 is the average BSA of an adult.

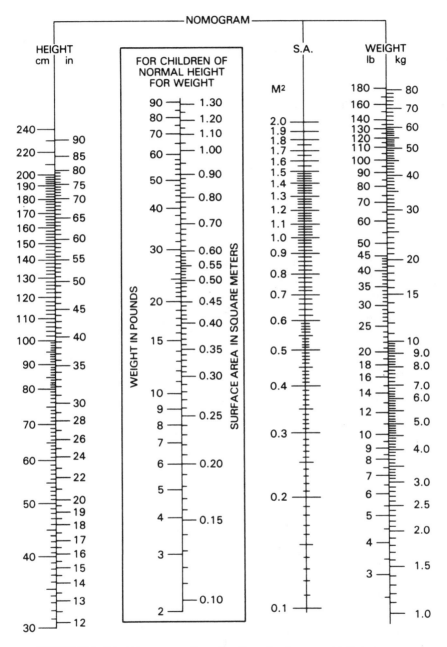

FIGURE 11.8. West Nomogram (for estimation of surface areas). Surface area is indicated where a straight line connecting height and weight intersects surface area (S.A.) column, or if patient is approximately of normal proportion, from weight alone (enclosed area). *(Nomogram modified from data of E. Boyd by C.D. West; from Behrman RE (ed): Nelson Textbook of Pediatrics, 14th ed. Philadelphia: Saunders, 1992, p. 1827.)*

18. Child's height: normal for weight.
    Child's weight: 28 lbs.
    Adult dose: 50–100 mg of drug.

    BSA:

    Child's dose:

19. Child's height: 26 inches.
    Child's weight: 4.3 kg.
    Adult dose: 0.5 mg per dose.

    BSA:

    Child's Dose:

20. Child's height: normal for weight.
    Child's weight: 20 lbs.
    Adult dose: 0.5 Gm of drug.

    BSA:

    Child's dose:

21. Child's height: 21 inches.
    Child's weight: 8 pounds.
    Adult dose: 50 mg of drug.

    BSA:

    Child's dose:

22. Child's height: 120 cm.
    Child's weight: 23 kg.
    Adult dose: 500 mg of drug.

    BSA:

    Child's dose:

23. Child's height: 43 inches.
    Child's weight: 33 lbs.
    Adult dose: 1000 mg of drug.

    BSA:

    Child's dose:

24. Child's height: 140 cm.
    Child's weight: 110 lbs.
    Adult dose: gr x of a drug.

    BSA:

    Child's dose:

☐ Answers

17. BSA: 0.8

    Child's Dose: $\dfrac{0.8 \text{ BSA}}{1.7} \times 15 \text{ mg} = 7.05 \text{ or } 7 \text{ mg of the drug}$

18. BSA: 0.565

    Child's Dose: $\dfrac{0.565 \text{ BSA}}{1.7} \times 50 \text{ mg} = 16.6 \text{ mg}$

    OR

    $\dfrac{0.565 \text{ BSA}}{1.7} \times 100 \text{ mg} = 33.24 \text{ or } 33 \text{ mg}$

19. BSA: 0.285

    Child's Dose: $\dfrac{0.285 \text{ BSA}}{1.7} \times 0.5 \text{ mg} = 0.08 \text{ mg per dose}$

20. BSA: 0.45

    Child's Dose: $\dfrac{0.45 \text{ BSA}}{1.7} \times 0.5 \text{ Gm} = 0.132 \text{ Gm or } 132 \text{ mg}$

21. BSA = 0.24

    Child's Dose: $\dfrac{0.24}{1.7} \times 50 \text{ mg} = 7.05 \text{ or } 7 \text{ mg}$

22. BSA = 0.88

    Child's Dose: $\dfrac{0.88}{1.7} \times 500 \text{ mg} = 258.8 \text{ or } 259 \text{ mg}$

23. BSA = 0.66

$$\text{Child's Dose: } \frac{0.66}{1.7} \times 1000 \text{ mg} = 388 \text{ mg}$$

24. BSA = 1.46

$$\text{Child's Dose: } \frac{1.46}{1.7} \times 10 \text{ gr} = 8.6 \text{ or } 9 \text{ gr}$$

If you missed more than two problems in each area, review the section before starting the next chapter. Because this chapter requires use of formulas, make sure you are not making a math error.

Comprehensive Exam 1

Directions
The test is divided into sections and samples the content covered in the text. Take this test as you would a classroom exam. Limit your time on the test to 1½ to 2 hours. If you have mastered the content you should score 100%. Because the items are divided into sections, you will be able to identify areas of strength and areas that need additional work. Good Luck!

Abbreviations and Symbols

Match the abbreviation or symbol with the meaning.

a. a.c.	b. U	c. c̄	d. p.o.
e. s.o.s.	f. aa	g. supp	h. Rx
i. lb	j. NPO.	k. p.c.	l. ung
m. h.s.	n. caps	o. mEq	p. ʒ
q. O.D.	r. s.c.	s. ss	t. b.i.d.
u. tsp	v. gtt	w. ad lib	x. q.i.d.
y. ʒ	z. sol	aa. ℔	bb. O.U.
cc. amp	dd. O.S.	ee. s̄	

1. _____ of each

2. _____ nothing by mouth

3. _____ ointment

4. _____ drop

5. _____ pound

6. _____ after meals

7. _____ suppository

8. _____ one half

9. _____ take

10. _____ ampule

11. _____ milliequivalent

12. _____ capsule

13. _____ at bedtime

14. _____ as desired

15. _____ twice a day

16. _____ right eye

17. _____ ounce

18. _____ subcutaneous

19. _____ solution

20. _____ minim

21. _____ orally

22. _____ without

23. _____ once if necessary

24. _____ both eyes

25. _____ unit

Interpretation of Physician's Orders

26. Chloral hydrate gr viiss p.o. q h.s. p.r.n. for sleep. Take with ℥ viii fruit juice.

    a. What is the name of the medication?

    b. What is the prescribed dosage?

    c. How is the medication to be administered?

    d. When is the medication to be administered?

    e. What other directions are given?

27. Amikin® 15 mg per kg of body weight IV q.12.h.

    a. What is the name of the medication?

    b. What is the dosage to be administered?

    c. How is the medication to be administered?

    d. When is the medication to be administered?

28. Tr belladonna gtts xv and Amphojel® ℥ s̄s̄ qid p.o.

    a. What are the names of the medications?

    b. What is the prescribed dosage of each medication?

c. How is the medication to be administered?

d. When is the medication to be administered?

29. Mandol® 1 Gm IV piggyback q.6.h. Mix in 100 mL of 0.9% Sodium Chloride Solution.

   a. What are the names of the medications?

   b. What is the dosage of each medication?

   c. How are the medications to be administered?

   d. When are the medications to be administered?

   e. What other directions are given?

Interpretation of Labels

Identify the parts of the selected labels.

30.

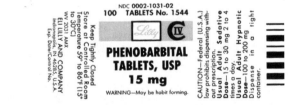

FIGURE 12.1.

   a. Drug name

   b. Drug form

   c. Dosage

   d. Manufacturer

   e. Number of tablets in container

   f. Storage directions

31.

Batch:
Expires:
Before reconstitution: Store below 86°F (30°C). After reconstitution with sterile water for injection, USP, store under refrigeration and use within 7 days. When stored at controlled room temperature, use within 48 hours.
821120
NDC 0026-8212-30
Mezlin®
Sterile mezlocillin sodium equivalent
to mezlocillin
Caution: Federal (USA) law prohibits dispensing without prescription
For IV or IM Use
MILES
For IV or IM Use
IV Use: Reconstitute with 20 mL sterile water for injection, USP, or other suitable diluent. SHAKE WELL. For infusion, dilute further to desired volume.
IM Use: Reconstitute with 8 mL sterile water for injection, USP, or 0.5% Lidocaine HCL injection, USP (without epinephrine). SHAKE WELL. Use within 24 hours.
For complete product information including dosage and administration, see accompanying package insert.

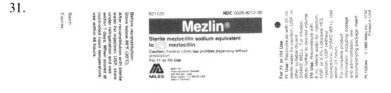

FIGURE 12.2.

a. Brand name

b. Generic name

c. Dosage

d. Drug administration routes

e. Reconstitution directions for IM administration

f. Manufacturer

32.

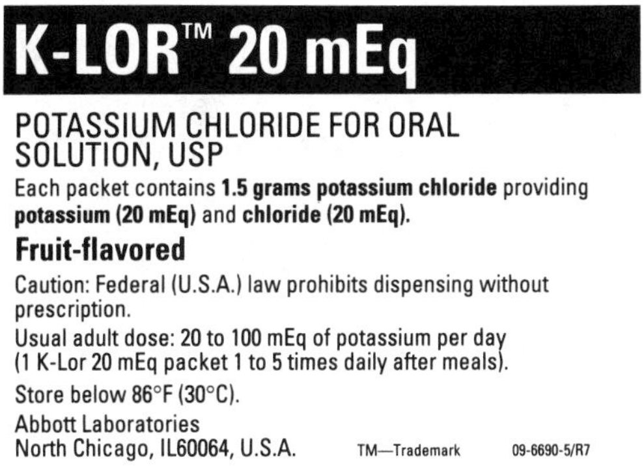
K-LOR™ 20 mEq
POTASSIUM CHLORIDE FOR ORAL SOLUTION, USP
Each packet contains 1.5 grams potassium chloride providing potassium (20 mEq) and chloride (20 mEq).
Fruit-flavored
Caution: Federal (U.S.A.) law prohibits dispensing without prescription.
Usual adult dose: 20 to 100 mEq of potassium per day (1 K-Lor 20 mEq packet 1 to 5 times daily after meals).
Store below 86°F (30°C).
Abbott Laboratories
North Chicago, IL60064, U.S.A.
TM—Trademark
09-6690-5/R7

FIGURE 12.3.

a. Brand name

b. Generic name

c. Dosage _____ mEq _____ grams

d. Drug form

e. Directions for preparation of drug for administration.

f. Manufacturer

33.

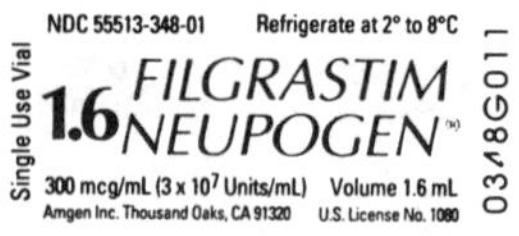

NDC 55513-348-01   Refrigerate at 2° to 8°C

1.6 *FILGRASTIM*
NEUPOGEN ™

Single Use Vial

300 mcg/mL (3 x 10⁷ Units/mL)   Volume 1.6 mL
Amgen Inc. Thousand Oaks, CA 91320   U.S. License No. 1080

0348G011

FIGURE 12.4.

a. Brand name

b. Generic name

c. Drug form

d. Dosage

e. Total mL in container

f. Drug container

g. Manufacturer

Calculation of Equivalents

34. 40 kg = _____ lbs

35. $\frac{1}{10}$ dram = _____ $\mathfrak{m}$

36. 0.1 mg = _____ gr

37. 270 mL = _____ oz

38. $\frac{1}{8}$ gr = _____ Gm

39. 12 $\mathfrak{m}$ = _____ cc

40. 800 μg = _____ mg

41. 5 dram = _____ mL

42. 4 tsp = _____ cc

43. $\frac{1}{120}$ gr = _____ mg

44. 3.5 pts = _____ mL

45. 35 mg = _____ Gm

46. $\frac{2}{3}$ oz = _____ tsp

47. 0.007 Gm = _____ μg

48. 1 cup _____ mL

Oral Medications

49. Order: Nizoral® (ketoconazole) gr v po daily.
Available: Nizoral 200 mg/scored tablets.

How many tablets should the patient receive?

50. Order: Naprosyn® (naproxen) 375 mg oral suspension q8h p.o.
    Available: Container of 475 mL of Naprosyn Suspension. Each
        5 mL contains 125 mg.

    a. How many tsp should the patient receive?

    b. If the patient received the first dose at 0800, what times will the
       next two doses be administered?

51. Order: Synthroid® (levothyroxine sodium) 0.1 mg p.o. daily.
    Available: Synthroid 300 μg per scored tablet and 200 μg per scored
        tablet.

    a. Which tablet should you use to compute the correct dose?

    b. How many or what portion of a tablet should you administer?

52. Order: Videx® (didanosine) tablets 0.3 Gm b.i.d.
    Available: Videx 100-mg and 150-mg tablets.

    Which tablet(s) and how many should the patient receive?

53. Order: Ceclor® (cefaclor) suspension 30 mg/kg/day.
    Available: Ceclor labeled as shown in Figure 12.5.

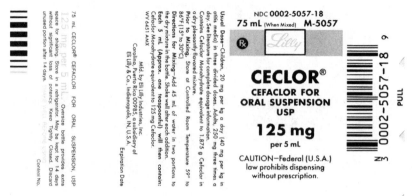

FIGURE 12.5.

Patient's weight: 77 lbs.

a. How should you prepare this new container of Ceclor?

b. After mixing, how many mL are in the container?

c. Identify the volume in mL that should be administered for each dose (Fig. 12.6).

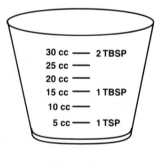

30 cc —	2 TBSP
25 cc —	
20 cc —	
15 cc —	1 TBSP
10 cc —	
5 cc —	1 TSP

FIGURE 12.6.

d. What are the directions for storage?

Parenteral Medications

54. Order: Levo-Dromoran® (levorphanol) 2.5 mg subcu q8h PRN pain.
    Available: 10-mL vial of Levo-Dromoran 2 mg/mL.

    Locate the volume in ℳ that you should administer (Fig. 12.7).

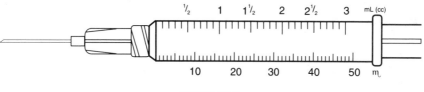

FIGURE 12.7.

55. Order: Inapsine® (droperidol) gr ¹⁄₁₀ IM on call to surgery.
    Available: 5-mL ampule labeled Inapsine 2.5 mg/mL.

    How many mL should you administer?

56. Order: Sublimaze® (fentanyl) 0.07 mg IM stat.
    Available: Sublimaze 2-mL ampule containing 50 mcg/mL.

    How many mL should the patient receive?

57. Order: Loxitane® IM (loxapine hydrochloride) 0.0125 Gm IM q6h.
    Available: 10-mL multidose vial, Loxitane 50 mg/mL.

    Locate the volume in mL that should be administered (Fig. 12.8).

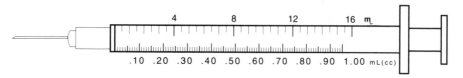

FIGURE 12.8.

58. Order: Adagen™ (pegademase bovine) 10 U/kg IM now.
    Available: 1.5-mL single-use vial of Adagen 250 U/mL.
    Patient's weight: 143 lbs.

    How many mL should the patient receive?

Reconstitution of Powders and Crystals

59. Order: Lupron Depot® (leuprolide acetate) 3.75 mg IM now.
    Available: Containers labeled as shown in Figure 12.9.

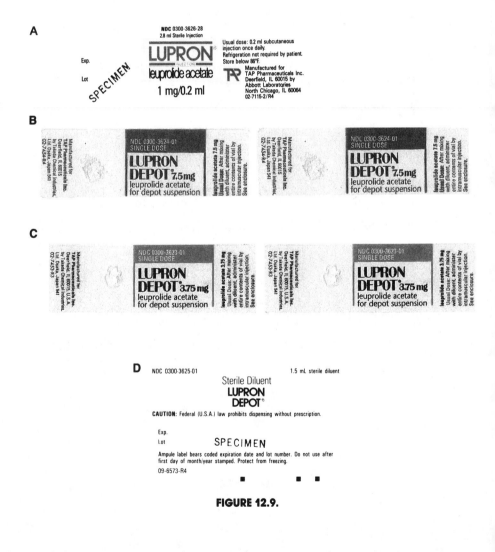

FIGURE 12.9.

a. Which vial should you select to use?

b. After adding the sterile diluent, how much should you administer?

60. Order: Cefotan® (cefotetan disodium) 500 mg q 12 h IM.
Available: A 1-Gm vial of Cefotan.
Use Table 12.1 to answer the questions that follow.

TABLE 12.1. Cefotan Reconstitution Table

For Intramuscular Use: Reconstitute with Sterile Water for Injection; Bacteriostatic Water for Injection; Normal Saline, USP; 0.5% Lidocaine HCl; or 1.0% Lidocaine HCl. Shake to dissolve and let stand until clear.

Vial Size	Amount of Diluent to Be Added (mL)	Approximate Withdrawable Vol (mL)	Approximate Average Concentration (mg/mL)
1 gram	2	2.5	400
2 gram	3	4.0	500

Copyright © PHYSICIANS' DESK REFERENCE® 1993 edition. Published by Medical Economics Data, Montvale, NJ 07645. Reprinted by permission. All rights reserved.

a. How many mL of diluent should you add to this 1-Gm vial?

b. Can 0.5% Lidocaine HCl be used as a diluent?

c. Locate the volume in minims you should administer to equal the prescribed dose (Fig. 12.10).

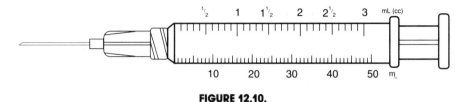

FIGURE 12.10.

61. Order: Leucovorin Calcium for Injection gr ⅕ IM q6h.
    Available: 50-mg vial of Leucovorin Calcium for Injection. Reconstitute with 5 mL of sterile diluent to yield 10 mg/mL.

    a. How many mL should you administer to equal the prescribed dose?

    b. How will you label the vial to define the prescribed dose per volume?

    c. What is the total reconstituted volume in this vial?

    d. The first dose will be given at 0600. Identify the remaining times in military time that the medication will be given during the 24-hour period.

Insulin

62. Order: Lente insulin U-100; 35 units ⎫
    Regular insulin U-100; 12 units ⎬ subq 7 a.m.

    Available: Insulins labeled as shown in Figure 12.11.

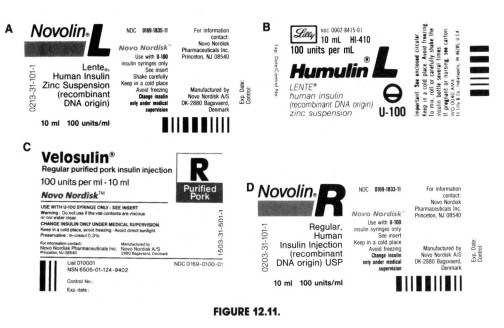

FIGURE 12.11.

a. Which insulins should you select and why?

b. Mark the correct dosage on the syringe shown in Figure 12.12.
Be sure and differentiate the amount of Regular and Lente.

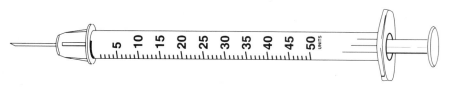

FIGURE 12.12.

c. If you only had a tuberculin syringe, how much should you administer?

63. Order: U-100 Humulin R ac and hs according to sliding scale. Blood
sugar 0600, 1100, 1630, and 2200.

Sliding Scale

Blood Sugar	Regular Insulin
↓ 120 mg/dL	0
121–180 mg/dL	2 units
181–240 mg/dL	6 units
241–300 mg/dL	10 units
301–360 mg/dL	12 units
↑ 360 mg/dL	call doctor

Indicate the number of units of Regular insulin you should administer for the following blood sugar results.

Time	Blood Sugar (mg/dL)	Insulin
0600	242	a. _____
1100	190	b. _____
1630	118	c. _____
2200	130	d. _____
	Total for day	e. _____

64. Order: Humulin® R 45 U s.c. stat.
    Available: Humulin R and the syringes shown in Figure 12.13.

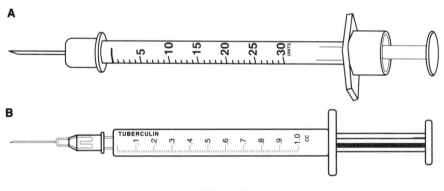

FIGURE 12.13.

Which syringe should you use and why?

65. Order: NPH 25 units and Regular 10 units a.c. q am.
    Available: NPH and Regular insulin and the syringes shown in Figure 12.14.

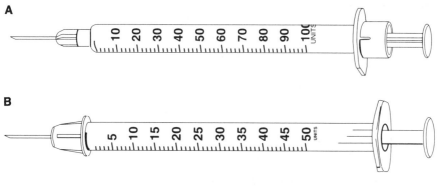

FIGURE 12.14.

Select the syringe that will give the most exact measurement and shade in the correct dose.

66. Your patient has an order for 55 units of $^{70}/_{30}$ Human Mixtard insulin s.c. stat.
    Available: The insulins labeled as shown in Figure 12.15.

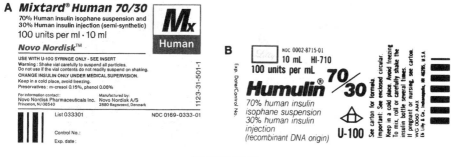

FIGURE 12.15.

The only syringe available is a tuberculin syringe.

a. Which insulin should you use and why?

b. How many mL should you administer?

Intravenous Fluids

67. Order: 250 mL of D$_5$W to run 12 hrs.
    Administration set: microdrop.

    What is the drop rate per minute?

68. Order: 1500 cc 5% D½ NS IV over 24 hrs.
    Administration set: 15 gtts/cc and 10 gtts/cc.

    Calculate the flow rate for *each* set.

    15 gtts/cc set

    10 gtts/cc set

69. Order: 1000 cc D$_5$RL to run at 65 cc/hr.
    Administration set: 20 gtts/cc.

    How fast should the IV run?

70. Mr. Smith's IV of 1000 cc D$_5$W c̄ 40 mEq KCl was started at 10 a.m.
    to run 8 hours. It is 2 p.m. and 650 cc remain in the bottle.
    Administration set: 15 gtts/mL

    a. At 10 a.m. the drop rate should have been set at _____ drops/min
       to infuse the fluid on time.

    b. How many cc should have infused by 2 p.m.?

    c. If you were to calculate the infusion rate for the fluid that re-
       mained at 2 p.m. to keep within the original 8-hour schedule, how
       fast should you set the IV?

71. You notice that the IV is dropping at 32 drops per minute. The IV
    administration set delivers 10 gtts/cc; 450 cc remain in the bottle. At
    this rate how many hours will it take to complete the infusion?

72. Order: 125 mg Solu-Medrol (methylprednisolone) IVPB q4h. Dissolve the drug in 50 cc of compatible solution and administer over 20 minutes.
    Administration set: 10 gtts/cc.

    For how many gtts/min should you regulate the IV?

73. Order: Ancef® (cefazolin sodium) 1 Gm IVPB q6h.
    Available: Ancef 1 Gm in 50 mL D5W to run at 100 cc/hr.
    Administration set: 20 gtts/mL.

    a. For how many drops per minute should you regulate the IV?

    b. The IV was started at 9 a.m. At this rate, what time should the IV be completed?

74. The physician has ordered 50 mEq of KCl (potassium chloride) to be added to 100 cc NS and administered at a rate of 10 mEq per hour.
    Administration set: microdrop.

    What should be the drop rate?

75. Order: Levophed® (norepinephrine bitartrate) 3 μg/min.
    Available: 500 cc D₅W with 1000 μg added.
    Administration set: 15 gtts/mL and a microdrop.

    Calculate the drop rate for *each* administration set.

    a. *15 gtts/cc set*

    b. *Microdrop*

    c. Which of the administration sets' flow rates would be easiest to count?

76. Order: Dobutrex® (dobutamine) IV at 20 mL/hr.
    Available: Dobutrex 500 mg in 500 mL D5W.
    Administration set: microdrop.

    How many mcg/min is the patient receiving?

77. Order: Tridil® (nitroglycerin) 10 mcg/min IV.
    Available: Tridil 5 mg in 250 mL D5W.

    a. What would the drop rate be with a microdrop?

    b. What would be the rate in mL/h?

78. You are using a Soluset and the IV is dripping at 17 gtts/min. The
    IV is 500 mL D5W with 25,000 U Heparin Sodium. How many units
    of Heparin is the patient receiving per hour?

79. Order: Aminophylline® (theophylline ethylenediamine) 25 mg per
    hour IV via electronic infusion device.
    Available: 500 mL D5W with 250 mg Aminophylline.

    How fast would you set the IV?

    For the following situations, determine the amount of time the IV
    should run if continued at the current drop rate.

	Current Drop Rate (gtts/min)	Administration Set (gtts/mL)	Fluid Left (mL)	Time (Hours and Minutes)
80.	33	10	150	

	Current Drop Rate (gtts/min)	Administration Set (gtts/mL)	Fluid Left (mL)	Time (Hours and Minutes)
81.	17	15	250	
82.	24	20	450	
83.	63	60	500	

84. Your IV of Levophed® (norepinephrine) 16 mg/500 cc D5W is infusing at a rate of 30 gtts/min.
Administration set: microdrop.

How many mcg/min and mg/h is the patient receiving?

85. Order: Aramine® (metaraminol bitartrate) 50 mg in 250 mL D5W to run at 60 μg/min.
Available: microdrop.

How fast should you set the IV?

86. Order: 1000 cc D5W with 40 mEq KCl, infuse at 8 mEq/h.
Administration set: 10 gtts/mL.

How fast should you regulate the IV?

87. Order: Cefizox® (ceftizoxine) 750 mg IV push q.8.h.
Available: Cefizox 1-Gm vial of powdered drug.
Directions for reconstitution: Add 10 mL of diluent for an approximate total volume of 10.7 mL.
Rate of administration: Administer over 4 minutes.

How many mL should you administer each minute _____ ; 30 seconds _____ ; and 15 seconds _____ ?

88. Order: Tazicef® (ceftazidime) 1 Gm IV push q8h. Administer through tubing over 3 to 5 minutes.
    Available: 1-Gm vial of powder. Add 3 mL of Sterile Water for Injection to achieve a concentration of 280 mg/mL.

    a. What is the total volume to be administered?

    b. What would be the rate of administration for the following times?

3 Minutes	5 Minutes
1 minute _____	1 minute _____
30 seconds _____	30 seconds _____
15 seconds _____	15 seconds _____

89. Your IV is dripping at 35 gtts/min. The administration set delivers 10 gtts/cc.
    Ordered: 1000 cc D5W with 40 mEq KCl IV.

    How many mEq of KCl is the patient receiving per hour?

Infants and Children

90. Order: Digoxin® (lanoxin) 0.035 mg po BID.
    Available: Digoxin Elixir 0.05 mg/mL.
    The recommended dose is 0.02 mg/kg/24 h.
    Child's weight: 9 lbs.

    a. How many mL equal the ordered dose?

b. Is this a safe dose for the child?

91. Ordered: Garamycin® (gentamicin sulfate) 44 mg IV TID.
    Available: Garamycin 20 mg per cc.
    Recommended dose: 5 to 7.5 mg/kg/day in 3 divided doses.
    Child's weight: 9 kg.

    a. How many cc equal the ordered dose?

    b. Is the present dose within the recommended dose range?

92. Order: Valium® (diazepam) 0.2 mg/kg IM × 1 dose.
    Available: Valium 5 mg/mL.
    Child's weight: 72 lbs.

    How many mL should you administer?

93. Order: Staphcillin® (methecillin sodium) 25 mg/kg/dose IV q8h.
    Available: Staphcillin 1-Gm vial. Add 1.5 mL of Sterile Water for
              Injection and each 1 mL will contain approximately 500
              mg Staphcillin.
    Child's weight: 4750 grams.

    a. What is the child's weight in kg?

    b. How many mL should you administer?

    Use the following formulas:

$$\frac{(4 \times \text{child's weight in kilograms}) + 7}{\text{Child's weight in kilograms} + 90} = \text{BSA in meters sq (m}^2)$$

$$\frac{\text{BSA}}{1.7} \times \text{Adult dose} = \text{Child's dose}$$

94. Jim weighs 20 lbs. The average adult dose of Keflin® (cephalothin sodium) is 4 Gm/24 hours.

    a. How much should Jim receive per 24 hours?

    b. The drug is ordered to be given q̄ 6 hr, and is available in 1 Gm/4 cc.

    How many cc should you administer per dose?

95. Order: Demerol® (meperidine hydrochloride) 25 mg IM stat.
    Available: Demerol 50 mg/mL.
    Child has a Body Surface Area of 0.70.
    Average adult dose is 50–100 mg.

    Is the ordered dose within the recommended amount?

96. Child's weight: 13.6 kg.
    Adult dose: Bicillin® C-R (procaine penicillin) 600,000 units daily.

    a. What is the maximum amount the child should receive?

    b. The doctor ordered 200,000 units divided into 4 equal doses. Was this within the safe range?

97. The average adult dose of Benadryl® (diphenhydramine HCl) is 100 mg/day divided into 4 equal doses.
    Child's weight: 75 lbs
    Available: Benadryl Elixir 5 mL contains 12.5 mg.

    a. How many mg should the child receive per dose?

b. How many mL should you administer per dose?

98. Order: Demerol® (meperidine) 15 mg IM q3h PRN pain.
Available: Demerol 25 mg/mL.
Child's weight: 25 kg.
Recommended dose for children is 0.5–0.8 mg per kg.

a. Is the ordered dose a safe dose?

b. What is the maximum dose for a child this size?

c. What is the volume you would administer to equal the order?

99. Order: A-Cillin® (amoxicillin for oral suspension) 250 mg q 6 hrs.
Available: A-Cillin 125 mg/5 mL oral suspension.
Recommended dose 20–40 mg/kg/day in divided doses q8h.
Child's weight: 18 kg.

a. What is the maximum and minimum individual dose?

b. What should you administer?

100. Order: Dycill® (dicloxacillin sodium) 125 mg po q6h.
Child's weight: 55 lbs.
Recommended dose: 12.5 mg/kg/day in evenly divided doses q 6 h.

a. What is the recommended individual dose?

b. Is the ordered dose a safe dose?

☐ **Answers**

Abbreviations and Symbols

1. f	2. j	3. l	4. v
5. i	6. k	7. g	8. s
9. h	10. cc	11. o	12. n
13. m	14. w	15. t	16. q
17. y	18. r	19. z	20. aa
21. d	22. ee	23. e	24. bb
25. b			

Interpretation of Physician's Orders

26. a. Chloral hydrate.
    b. Grains seven and one-half.
    c. By mouth.
    d. Whenever necessary for sleep every night at hour of sleep.
    e. The medication should be taken with eight ounces of fruit juice.
27. a. Amikin®.
    b. 15 milligrams per kilogram of body weight.
    c. Intravenously.
    d. Every 12 hours.
28. a. Tincture of belladonna and Amphojel®.
    b. 15 drops of tincture of belladonna and one-half ounce of Amphojel.
    c. By mouth.
    d. Four times a day.
29. a. Mandol and 0.9% Sodium Chloride Solution.
    b. 1 gram of Mandol and 100 milliliters of 0.9% Sodium Chloride Solution.
    c. Intravenous by piggyback.
    d. Every 6 hours.
    e. The Mandol is to be diluted in 100 milliliters of 0.9% Sodium Chloride Solution.

Interpretation of Labels

30. a. Phenobarbital.
    b. Tablets.
    c. 15 mg/tablet.
    d. Eli Lilly and Co.
    e. 100 tablets.
    f. Room temperature 59 to 86°F. Keep tightly closed.

31. a. Mezlin®.
    b. Meziocillin sodium.
    c. 2 grams.
    d. IV or IM.
    e. Add 8 mL Sterile Water for Injection or 0.5% Lidocaine HCl for Injection (without epinephrine).
    f. Miles.
32. a. K-LOR®.
    b. Potassium Chloride.
    c. 20 mEq, 1.5 Gm.
    d. Powder.
    e. Place one packet into glass and add 4 ounces cold water or juice. Stir until dissolved.
    f. Abbott Laboratories.
33. a. Neupogen®.
    b. Filgrastim.
    c. Liquid.
    d. 300 mcg/mL.
    e. 1.6 mL.
    f. Single-use vial.
    g. Amgen, Inc.

Calculation of Equivalents

34. 1 kg : 2.2 lbs :: 40 kg : X lbs

$$1 \ X = 88 \ lbs$$

35. 1 dr : 60 $\mathfrak{m}$ :: $\frac{1}{10}$ dr : X $\mathfrak{m}$

$$1 \ X = 6 \ \mathfrak{m} \ (\mathfrak{m} \ vi)$$

36. 1 mg : $\frac{1}{60}$ gr :: 0.1 mg : X gr

$$1 \ X = \frac{1}{10} \times \frac{1}{60}$$

$$X = \frac{1}{600} \ gr$$

(if equivalent 1000 mg : 15 gr, $X = \frac{1}{666}$ gr)

37. 30 mL : 1 oz :: 270 mL : X oz

$$30 \ X = 270$$

$$X = 9 \ (\text{\textzoz}ix)$$

38. 15 gr : 1 Gm :: $\frac{1}{8}$ gr : X Gm

$$15 \ X = \frac{1}{8}$$

$$X = \frac{1}{120} \ or \ 0.0083 \ Gm$$

(if equivalent 1 gr : 0.06 Gm, X = 0.0075 Gm)

39. 16 ℥ : 1 cc :: 12 ℥ : X cc

    16 X = 12

    X = 0.75 cc

40. 1000 μg : 1 mg :: 800 μg : X mg

    1000 X = 800

    X = 0.8 mg

41. 1 dr : 4 mL :: 5 dr : X mL

    1 X = 20 mL

42. 1 tsp : 5 mL :: 4 tsp : X cc

    1 X = 20 cc

43. 1 gr : 60 mg :: $\frac{1}{120}$ gr : X mg

    1 X = $\frac{60}{120}$

    X = 0.5 mg

(if equivalent 15 gr : 1000 mg, X = 0.55 mg

44. 1 pt : 500 mL :: 3.5 pts : X mL

    1 X = 1750 mL

45. 1000 mg : 1 Gm :: 35 mg : X Gm

    1000 X = 35

    X = 0.035 Gm

46. ½ oz : 3 tsp :: ⅔ oz : X tsp

    ½ X = $\frac{6}{3}$

    X = 4 tsp

47. 1 Gm : 1000 mg :: 0.007 Gm : X mg

    1 X = 7 mg

    1 mg : 1000 μg :: 7 mg : X μg

    1 X = 7000 μg

48. 8 oz = 1 cup

    1 oz : 30 mL :: 8 oz : X mL

    1 X = 240 mL

Oral Medications

49. 1 gr : 60 mg :: 5 gr : X mg

    1 X = 300 mg

    200 mg : 1 tab :: 300 mg : X tab

    200 X = 300

    X = 1.5 tab

50. a. 5 mL = 1 tsp

    125 mg : 1 tsp :: 375 mg : X tsp

    125 X = 375

    X = 3 tsp

    b. 1600 and 2400

51. a. The 200 μg tablet

    b. 200 μg : 1 tab :: 100 μg : X tablets

    200 X = 100

    X = ½ tablet

52. 1 Gm : 1000 mg :: 0.3 Gm : X mg

    1 X = 300 mg

    150 mg : 1 tab :: 300 mg : X tab

    150 X = 300

    X = 2 tabs of the 150-mg tablet

    Reduces the number of tablets the patient is to take.

53. a. Add 45 mL of water in two portions to the dry mixture (eg, 22 mL, then 23 mL). Shake well after each addition.

    b. 75 mL

c. 2.2 lbs : 1 kg :: 77 lbs : X kg

$$2.2 \ X = 77$$

$$X = 35 \ kg$$

30 mg : 1 kg :: X mg : 35 kg

$$1 \ X = 1050 \ mg/day$$

$$1050 \ mg \div 3 \ doses = 350 \ mg/dose$$

125 mg : 5 mL :: 350 mg : X mL

$$125 \ X = 1750$$

$$X = 14 \ mL$$

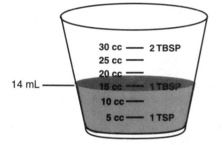

14 mL

For a more accurate measurement, use a 20-mL syringe to prepare the correct amount. Then place the 14 mL in the medication container.

FIGURE 12.16.

d. Store in refrigerator. May be kept 14 days. Keep tightly closed.

Parenteral Medications

54.

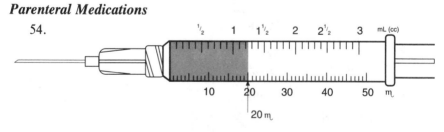

FIGURE 12.17.

2 mg : 16 ♏ :: 2.5 mg : X ♏

$$2 \ X = 40$$

$$X = 20 \ ♏$$

55. 60 mg : 1 gr :: X mg : gr ¹⁄₁₀

$$1 \ X = {}^{60}\!/_{10} = 6 \ mg$$

2.5 mg : 1 mL :: 6 mg : X mL

2.5 X = 6

X = 2.4 mL

56. 1000 mcg : 1 mg :: X mcg : 0.07 mg

1 X = 70 mcg

50 mcg : 1 mL :: 70 mcg : X mL

50 X = 70

X = 1.4 mL

57.

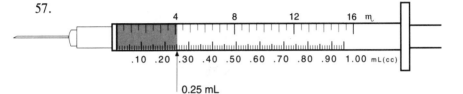

0.25 mL

FIGURE 12.18.

1000 mg : 1 Gm :: X mg : 0.0125 Gm

1 X = 12.5 mg

50 mg : 1 mL :: 12.5 mg : X mL

50 X = 12.5

X = 0.25 mL

58. 2.2 lbs : 1 kg :: 143 lbs : X kg

2.2 X = 143

X = 65 kg

10 U : 1 kg :: X U : 65 kg

1 X = 650 U

250 U : 1 mL :: 650 U : X mL

250 X = 650

X = 2.6 mL

Withdraw 1.5 mL from first vial   = 375 mg
Withdraw 1.1 mL from second vial = 275 mg
        2.6 mL   650 mg

Reconstitution of Powders and Crystals

59. a. C, the 3.75-mg vial of Lupron Depot.

    b. Entire contents of vial.

60. a. 2 mL

    b. Yes

    c. 400 mg : 16 ℔ :: 500 mg : X ℔

    $$400 \text{ X} = 8000$$

    $$\text{X} = 20 \text{ ℔}$$

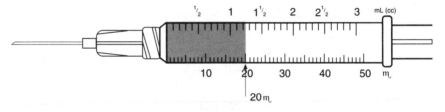

FIGURE 12.19.

61. a. 60 mg : 1 gr :: X mg : gr ⅕

    $$1 \text{ X} = {}^{60}\!/_5$$

    $$\text{X} = 12 \text{ mg}$$

    10 mg : 1 mL :: 12 mg : X mL

    $$10 \text{ X} = 12$$

    $$\text{X} = 1.2 \text{ mL}$$

    b. 12 mg/1.2 mL

    c. 10 mg : 1 mL :: 50 mg : X mL

    $$10 \text{ X} = 50$$

    $$\text{X} = 5 \text{ mL}$$

    d. 1200; 1800; 2400

Insulin

62. a. Novolin L and Novolin R. They both have same manufacturer and source (human).

b.

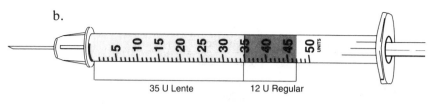

35 U Lente   12 U Regular

FIGURE 12.20.

   c. 0.47 mL on a tuberculin syringe.

63. Sliding Scale results: 0600 = 10 units; 1100 = 6 units; 1630 = 0 units; 2200 = 2 units; for a total of 18 units for the day.

64. Select the tuberculin syringe (1 cc). The order is for more than would fit into the U-100 $\frac{3}{10}$th or 30-unit syringe. You would withdraw 0.45 cc of Humulin R.

65. The 50 unit per $\frac{1}{2}$ cc will give the most exact measure, because it is measured in single units and 35 units can easily be measured. The U-100 syringe would require you to approximate the 35 units as the markings are at 34 and 36 units.

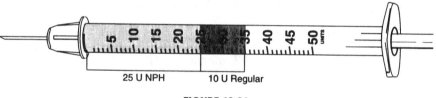

25 U NPH   10 U Regular

FIGURE 12.21.

66. You should use the Mixtard Human $^{70}/_{30}$ because the order specifically requested that brand even though the other brand was also $^{70}/_{30}$.

Using a tuberculin syringe you should administer 0.55 mL.

Intravenous Fluids

67. $\dfrac{250 \text{ mL}}{12 \text{ hours}}$ = 20.8 cc/h

   21 gtts/min

   Remember gtts/min and cc/h are same with microdrop.

68. *15 gtts/cc set*

$$\frac{1500 \text{ cc}}{24 \text{ hours}} \times \frac{15 \text{ gtts/cc}}{60 \text{ minutes}} = 15.6 \text{ or } 16 \text{ gtts/min}$$

10 gtts/cc set

$$\frac{1500 \text{ cc}}{24 \text{ hours}} \times \frac{10 \text{ gtts/cc}}{60 \text{ minutes}} = 10.4 \text{ or } 10 \text{ gtts/min}$$

69. $\dfrac{65 \text{ cc}}{1 \text{ hour}} \times \dfrac{20 \text{ gtts/cc}}{60 \text{ min}} = 21 \text{ gtts/min}$

70. a. $\dfrac{1000 \text{ cc}}{8 \text{ hours}} \times \dfrac{15 \text{ gtts/cc}}{60 \text{ min}} = 31.25 \text{ or } 31 \text{ gtts/min}$

    b. 500 cc (125 cc/hour × 4 hours)

    c. $\dfrac{650 \text{ cc}}{4 \text{ hours}} \times \dfrac{15 \text{ gtts/cc}}{60 \text{ minutes}} = 40.6 \text{ or } 41 \text{ gtts/min}$

71. 32 gtts/min ÷ 10 gtts/cc = 3.2 cc/min

    450 cc ÷ 3.2 cc/min = 140.625 min or 2 hours 21 minutes

72. $\dfrac{50\text{cc}}{20 \text{ minutes}} \times 10 \text{ gtts/cc} = 25 \text{ gtts/min}$

73. a. $\dfrac{100 \text{ cc}}{60 \text{ minutes}} \times 20 \text{ gtts/cc} = 33.33 \text{ or } 33 \text{ gtts/min}$

    b. 9:30 a.m.

$$100 \text{ cc} : 60 \text{ minutes} :: 50 \text{ cc} : X \text{ min}$$
$$100 \, X = 3000$$
$$X = 30 \text{ minutes}$$

74. 10 mEq = 20 cc

$$\frac{20 \text{ cc}}{60 \text{ minutes}} \times 60 \text{ gtts/mL} = 20 \text{ gtts/min}$$

75. a. *15 gtts/cc set*

$$1000 \text{ μg} : 500 \text{ cc} :: 3 \text{ μg} : X \text{ cc}$$
$$1000 \, X = 1500$$
$$X = 1.5 \text{ cc}$$
$$1.5 \text{ cc} \times 15 \text{ gtts} = 22.5 \text{ or } 23 \text{ gtts/min}$$

    b. *Microdrop*

$$1.5 \text{ cc} = 3 \text{ μg}$$
$$1.5 \text{ cc} \times 60 \text{ gtts/cc} = 90 \text{ gtts/min}$$

c. Probably the 23 gtts/min with the 15 gtts/mL set would be the easiest to count, but the microdop might be safer because Levophed is a powerful medication and a smaller dose at one time is easier to counteract or follow for results or side effects. Use the one that would allow for fewest errors.

76. 500 mg = 500,000 mcg

500,000 mcg : 500 mL :: X mcg : 20 mL

$$500 \text{ X} = 10,000,000$$

$$\text{X} = 20,000 \text{ mcg/20 mL}$$

20,000 mcg : 1 hour (60 minutes) :: X mcg : 1 minute

$$60 \text{ X} = 20,000$$

$$\text{X} = 333.33 \text{ mcg/min}$$

77. a. 5 mg = 5000 mcg

5000 mcg : 250 mL :: 10 mcg : X mL

$$5000 \text{ X} = 2500$$

$$\text{X} = 0.5 \text{ mL/min} \times 60 \text{ gtts/mL} = 30 \text{ gtts/min}$$

b. 0.5 mL : 1 min :: X mL : 60 minutes

$$\text{X} = 30 \text{ mL/h}$$

78. 17 gtts : X mL :: 60 gtts : 1 mL

$$60 \text{ X} = 17$$

$$\text{X} = 0.28 \text{ mL/min} \times 60 \text{ minutes} = 16.9 \text{ or } 17 \text{ cc/h}$$

500 mL : 25,000 U :: 17 mL : X U

$$500 \text{ X} = 425,000$$

$$\text{X} = 850 \text{ U Heparin/h}$$

79. 500 mL : 250 mg :: X mL : 25 mg

$$250 \text{ X} = 12,500$$

$$\text{X} = 50 \text{ mL/h}$$

80. $\dfrac{150 \text{ mL}}{\text{Time (X)}} \times \dfrac{10 \text{ gtts/mL}}{60 \text{ minutes}} = 33 \text{ gtts/min}$

$$\text{X} = \frac{150 \times 10}{33 \times 60} = 0.75 \text{ hours} \times 60 = 45 \text{ minutes}$$

81. $\dfrac{250 \text{ mL}}{\text{Time (X)}} \times \dfrac{15 \text{ gtts/mL}}{60 \text{ minutes}} = 17 \text{ gtts/min}$

$X = \dfrac{250 \times 15}{17 \times 60} = 3.67 \text{ or } 3 \text{ hours } 40 \text{ minutes} (3.7 = 3 \text{ h } 42 \text{ minutes})$

82. $\dfrac{450 \text{ mL}}{\text{Time (X)}} \times \dfrac{20 \text{ gtts/mL}}{60 \text{ minutes}} = 24 \text{ gtts/min}$

$X = \dfrac{450 \times 20}{24 \times 60} = 6.25 \text{ or } 6 \text{ hours } 15 \text{ minutes} (6.3 = 6 \text{ h } 18 \text{ minutes})$

83. $\dfrac{500 \text{ mL}}{\text{Time (X)}} \times \dfrac{60 \text{ gtts/mL}}{60 \text{ min}} = 63 \text{ gtts/min}$

$X = \dfrac{500 \times 60}{63 \times 60} = 7.9 \text{ or } 7 \text{ hours and } 54 \text{ minutes}$

84. 16,000 mcg : 500 cc :: X mcg : 1 cc

$$500 \text{ X} = 16,000$$

$$X = 32 \text{ mcg/mL}$$

32 mcg : 60 gtts :: X mcg : 30 gtts

$$60 \text{ X} = 960$$

$$X = 16 \text{ mcg/min}$$

16 mcg/min $\times$ 60 minutes = 960 mcg/h = 0.96 mg/h

85. 50,000 mcg : 250 mL :: X mcg : 1 mL

$$250 \text{ X} = 50,000$$

$$X = 200 \text{ mcg/mL}$$

200 mcg : 60 gtts :: 60 mcg : X gtts

$$200 \text{ X} = 3600$$

$$X = 18 \text{ gtts/min}$$

86. 40 mEq : 1000 cc :: 8 mEq : X cc

$$40 \text{ X} = 8000$$

$$X = 200 \text{ cc/h}$$

$\dfrac{200 \text{ cc}}{1 \text{ hour}} \times \dfrac{10 \text{ gtts/cc}}{60 \text{ minutes}} = 33.33 \text{ or } 33 \text{ gtts/min}$

87. 1000 mg : 10.7 mL : : 750 mg : X mL

    1000 X = 8025

    X = 8.025 = 8 mL total volume

    8 mL over 4 minutes, 2 mL per 1 minute, 1 mL per 30 seconds, and 0.5 mL per 15 seconds.

88. a. 280 mg : 1 mL : : 1000 mg : X mL

    280 X = 1000

    X = 3.57 or 3.6 mL total volume

    b. *3 minutes*

    1 minute = 1.2 mL, 30 seconds = 0.6 mL, and 15 seconds = 0.3 mL.

    5 minutes

    1 minute = 0.72 mL, 30 seconds = 0.36 or 0.4 mL, and 15 seconds = 0.18 or 0.2 mL.

89. 1000 cc : 40 mEq : : 1 cc : X mEq

    1000 X = 40

    X = 0.04 mEq/cc

    0.04 mEq : 10 gtts/mL : : X mEq : 35 gtts/min

    10 X = 1.4

    X = 0.14 mEq/min × 60 minutes

    = 8.4 mEq/h

Infants and Children

90. 9 lbs = 4.09 kg

    a. Ordered Dose:

    0.05 mg: 1 mL : : 0.035 mg : X mL

    0.05 X = 0.035

    X = 0.7 mL per ordered dose

    b. Recommended Dose:

    0.02 mg × 4.09 kg = 0.0818 or 0.082 mg/24 hours

    Divided into 2 doses (BID) = 0.041 mg per dose

    Ordered dose is a safe dose.

91. a. 20 mg : 1 cc :: 44 mg : X cc

    20 X = 44

    X = 2.2 cc per dose

  b. Recommended:

    5 mg × 9 kg = 45 mg/day ÷ 3 = 15 mg per dose

    7.5 mg × 9 kg = 67.5 mg/day ÷ 3 = 22.5 mg/dose

    Ordered: 44 mg/dose exceeds the recommended individual dosage and the total (44 mg × 3[TID]) 132 mg/day exceeds the recommended daily dose. This is not within the dosage range.

92. 72 lbs = 32.73 kg

    0.2 mg × 32.73 kg = 6.55 mg per dose

    5 mg : 1 mL :: 6.55 mg : X mL

    5 X = 6.55

    X = 1.31 or 1.3 mL

93. a. 1000 Gm : 1 kg :: 4750 Gm : X kg

    1000 X = 4750

    X = 4.75 kg

  b. 25 mg × 4.75 kg = 118.75 mg or 119 mg per dose

    500 mg : 1 mL :: 119 mg : X mL

    X = 0.238 = 0.24 mL of the drug

94. a. $\dfrac{(4 \times 9.09 \text{ kg}) + 7}{9.09 + 90} = \dfrac{43.36}{99.09} = 0.4375 = 0.44 \text{ BSA}$

    $\dfrac{0.44 \text{ BSA}}{1.7} \times 4 \text{ Gm} = 1.035 \text{ Gm/24 hours}$

  b. 0.259 Gm/dose (1.035 Gm ÷ 4 doses)

    0.259 Gm : X cc :: 1 Gm : 4 cc

    X = 1.036 or 1 cc per dose

95. 50 mg adult (minimum)

    $\dfrac{0.7 \text{ BSA}}{1.7} \times 50 \text{ mg} = 20.58 \text{ mg}$

100 mg adult (maximum)

$$\frac{0.7 \text{ BSA}}{1.7} \times 100 \text{ mg} = 41.17 \text{ mg}$$

Yes—25 mg falls between 20.58 mg and 41.17 mg

96. a. $\dfrac{(4 \times 132.6) + 7}{13.6 + 90} = \dfrac{61.4}{103.6} = 0.59 \text{ BSA}$

   $\dfrac{0.59 \text{ BSA}}{1.7} \times 600,000 \text{ units} = 208,235 \text{ units}$

   b. Yes

97. 75 lbs = 34.1 kg

   a. $\dfrac{(4 \times 34.1) + 7}{34.1 + 90} = \dfrac{143.4}{124.1} = 1.155 \text{ or } 1.16 \text{ BSA M}^2$

   $\dfrac{1.16 \text{ BSA}}{1.7} \times 100 = 68.24 \text{ mg/day} \div 4 = 17.06 \text{ mg/dose}$

   b. 12.5 mg : 5 mL :: 17 mg : X mL

   $$12.5 \text{ X} = 85$$

   $$\text{X} = 6.8 \text{ mL}$$

98. a. Ordered dose within the safe recommended range.

   b. 0.8 mg × 25 kg = 20 mg per dose

   c. 15 mg : X mL :: 25 mg : 1 mL

   $$25 \text{ X} = 15$$

   $$\text{X} = 0.6 \text{ mL}$$

99. a. Maximum: 40 mg × 18 kg = 720 mg/day ÷ 3 (q8h) = 240 mg

   Minimum: 20 mg × 18 kg = 360 mg/day ÷ 3 (q8h) = 120 mg

   b. You should not administer the drug until order clarified.

   The order for 250 mg per dose is slightly higher than the maximum 240 mg per dose; but the order is for q 6 h, which would make the total for 24 hours 1000 mg, which greatly exceeds the recommended dose.

100. a. 55 lbs = 25 kg

   12.5 mg × 25 kg = 312.5 mg/day ÷ 4 = 78.125 or 78 mg/dose

   b. Ordered dose is 125 mg per dose. This is not a safe dose. You should notify the physician before proceeding.

Comprehensive Exam 2

Directions

The test is divided into sections and samples the content covered in the text. Take this test as you would a classroom exam. Limit your time on the test to 2 hours. If you have mastered the content you should score 100%. Because the items are divided into sections you will be able to identify areas of strength and areas that need additional work.

Interpretation of Labels

Identify the parts of the selected labels.

1.

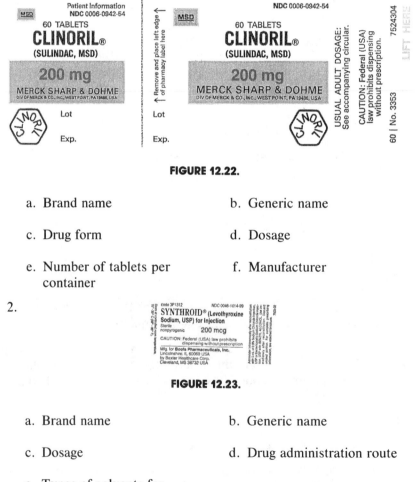

FIGURE 12.22.

a. Brand name

b. Generic name

c. Drug form

d. Dosage

e. Number of tablets per container

f. Manufacturer

2.

SYNTHROID® (Levothyroxine Sodium, USP) for Injection
Sterile nonpyrogenic   200 mcg

FIGURE 12.23.

a. Brand name

b. Generic name

c. Dosage

d. Drug administration route

e. Types of solvents for reconstitution

f. Amount of diluent   g. Storage directions

3.

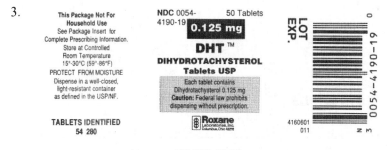

This Package Not For
Household Use
See Package Insert for
Complete Prescribing Information.
Store at Controlled
Room Temperature
15°-30°C (59°-86°F)
PROTECT FROM MOISTURE
Dispense in a well-closed,
light-resistant container
as defined in the USP/NF.

TABLETS IDENTIFIED
54 280

NDC 0054-   50 Tablets
4190-19

0.125 mg

DHT ™

DIHYDROTACHYSTEROL
Tablets USP

Each tablet contains
Dihydrotachysterol 0.125 mg
Caution: Federal law prohibits
dispensing without prescription.

Roxane
Laboratories, Inc.
Columbus, Ohio 43216

4160601
011

LOT
EXP.

0054-4190-19

FIGURE 12.24.

a. Brand name   b. Generic name

c. Drug form   d. Dosage

e. Number of tablets per   f. Manufacturer
   container

Calculation of Equivalents

4. 0.080 Gm = _____ mg

5. ¾ oz = _____ drams

6. ¹⁄₁₀₀ gr = _____ mg

7. ⅛ tsp = _____ ℳ

8. 6.5 mg = _____ µg

9. 2½ glasses = _____ ml

10. 33 lbs = _____ kg

11. 5.5 tbsp = _____ oz

12. 0.02 Gm = _____ gr

13. 0.45 mL = _____ ℳ

14. 300 mg = _____ gr

15. $3\frac{1}{3}$ tsp   = _____ mL

16. 1750 mg   = _____ Gm

17. 4.2 drams = _____ mL

18. 4 gr   = _____ Gm

Oral Medications

19. Order: Cefzil® (cefprozil) oral suspension 500 mg po q 12 h.
    Available: Cefzil oral suspension 125 mg/5 mL.

    a. Mark the volume in mL that should be administered (Fig. 12.25)

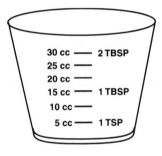

FIGURE 12.25.

    b. The first dose is given at 0900. When is the next dose due?

20. Order: K-tab® (Potassium Chloride) 1.5 Gm p.o. q.d.
    Available: The container labeled as shown in Figure 12.26.

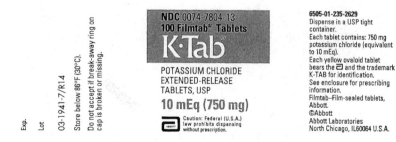

a. How many tablets should the patient receive?

b. How would you describe what the K-tab tablet looks like to the patient?

c. How many mEq is the patient receiving per day?

21. Order: Symmetrel® (amantadine hydrochloride) syrup 0.1 g b.i.d. p.o.
    Available: Symmetrel syrup 50 mg/5 mL.

    Locate amount in tsp that the patient should receive (Fig. 12.27).

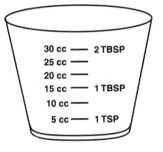

FIGURE 12.27.

22. Order: Nolvadex® (tamoxifen citrate) gr ⅓ po bid.
    Available: Nolvadex 10 mg/tablet.

    a. How many tablets should you administer?

    b. The recommended daily dose is 0.4–0.8 mg/kg. Is this 121-lb patient receiving a dose that is within this recommended range?

23. Order: Hivid® (zalcitabine) 750 mcg po q8h.
    Available: 0.375 mg/tablet.

    How many tablets should the patient receive?

Parenteral Medications

24. Order: Antilirium® (physostigmine salicylate) 550 mcg IM stat.
    Available: Antilirium ampule 1 mg/mL.

    Locate the volume in mL that should be administered.

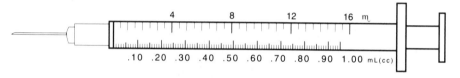

FIGURE 12.28.

25. Order: Furosemide 25 mg IM @ 10 a.m.
    Available:

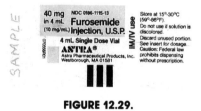

FIGURE 12.29.

a. How many mL should the patient receive?

b. How many mg of Furosemide are in this container?

c. This drug is in what kind of container?

d. What is the route of administration of this drug?

26. Order: Urecholine® (benthanechol chloride) gr 1/20 subc NOW.
    Available: Urecholine vial labeled 5 mg/mL.

    How many ℳ of Urecholine should you administer?

27. Order: Levsin® (hyoscyamine sulfate) 5 μg/kg of body weight IM on
    call to surgery.
    Available: Ampule labeled Levsin 0.5 mg/mL.
    Patient's weight: 99 lbs.

    a. How many μg of Levsin was ordered?

    b. How many mL of Levsin (_____ μg/mL) should you administer?

28. Order: Toradol® (ketorolac tromethamine) 25 mg q6h IM.
    Available: Toradol 30 mg/mL in a prefilled syringe.

    a. How many mL should you administer?

    b. How many mL should you expel from the syringe?

Reconstitution of Powders and Crystals

29. Order: Rocephin® (ceftraiaxone sodium) 1.5 g in equally divided doses
    q 12 h deep IM.
    Available: 1-g vial of Rocephin. Add 3.6 mL of diluent to the 1-g vial
    to yield 250 mg/mL.

a. How many mL of diluent should you add to the vial?

b. How many mL should you administer per each dose?

30. Order: Desferal® (deferoxamine mesylate) 750 mg IM q day.
    Available: Desferal 500-mg vial. Add 2 mL of Sterile Water for Injection to yield 250 mg/mL.

    Describe how you should prepare the vial(s) of Desferal.

    How many mL should you administer to equal the prescribed dose?

31. Order: Unipen® (nafcillin sodium) 500 mg I.M. q.6.h.
    Available: Unipen 2-Gm vial. Following reconstitution, the vial should be used within 3 days if kept at room temperature.

Unipen Reconstitution Table

Vial Size	Amount of Diluent (mL)	Nafcillin Sodium Solution (mL)
500 mg	1.7	2
1 Gm	3.4	4
2 Gm	6.8	8

a. How many mL of diluent should you add to the 2-Gm vial?

b. How many mL of Unipen should you administer?

c. What is the amount of displacement in the 2-Gm vial?

d. You reconstituted this vial June 2 at 6 a.m. When should the vial be discarded?

Insulin

32. Order: 32 units of Mixtard® Human 70/30 U-100 at 0700.
    Available: U-100 Mixtard Human 70/30 10-mL vial and syringe shown in Figure 12.30.

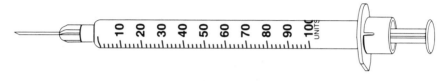

FIGURE 12.30.

a. Shade the syringe with the amount of insulin you should administer.

b. If you did not have an insulin syringe, what syringe would be appropriate?

c. How many mL should you administer?

33. Order: Novulin® R insulin s.c. ac per sliding scale.

Sliding Scale

Blood Sugar (mL/dL)	Units of Insulin
0–150	0
151–250	8
251–350	13
351–400	18
> 400	call physician

At 0730 the patient's blood sugar is 275. How much insulin should you administer?

Mark the dosage on the appropriate syringe (Fig. 12.31).

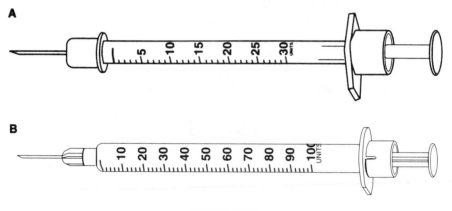

FIGURE 12.31.

34. Order: Blood glucose by finger stick each AM and at time of evening meal. U-100 Novolin® R according to sliding scale. U-100 Novolin L 25 units before breakfast and 18 units before evening meal.

Sliding Scale

Blood Sugar (mg/dL)	Regular Insulin (units)
↓ 60	5
60–120	6
121–200	7
201–300	8
↑ 300	9

At 7:00 a.m. blood sugar 90 mg/dL
6:00 p.m. blood sugar 240 mg/dL

a. How many units Novolin R and Novolin L should you administer before breakfast?

b. What is the total number of units of insulin (Novolin R and Novolin L) for the day?

35. Order: U-100 Humulin® N; 42 units ⎱ subc 6:30 am daily
           U-100 Humulin® R; 7 units ⎰
   Available: U-100 Humulin N and U-100 Humulin R insulin
            U-100 1-cc insulin syringe
            U-100 Lo-Dose insulin syringe

a. What is the total number of units to be administered at 6:30 a.m.?

b. Which insulin syringe should you use?

c. If an insulin syringe were not available what should you use?

d. How many mL to the nearest hundredth should you administer?

Humulin N _____ mL

Humulin R _____ mL

Total _____ mL

Intravenous Fluids and Medications

36. Order: 500 cc of D5W to run 12 hours.
Administration set: 15 gtts/mL.

What is the drop per minute?

37. Order: 1000 cc D5NS to run at 75 cc/h.
Administration set: 10 gtts/mL.

How fast should you regulate the drop rate?

38. Mr. Jones' IV of 1000 cc NS with 1 amp. multivitamin was started at 7 a.m. to run 6 hours. It is 11:00 a.m. and 450 cc remain in the bag. Administration set: 20 gtts/mL.

   a. At 7 a.m. the drop rate should have been set at _____ drops/min to infuse the fluid on time.

   b. How many cc should have infused by 11:00 a.m.?

   c. If you were to calculate the infusion rate for the fluid that remained at 11:00 a.m. to keep the original 6-hour schedule, how fast should you set the IV?

39. You notice that the IV is dropping at 26 drops per minute. The IV administration set delivers 15 gtts/mL; 450 cc remain in the bag.

   a. How many cc per minute is the IV infusing at the present rate?

   b. How long in hours and minutes will it take to infuse the remaining fluid at the current rate?

40. Order: Levophed® (levarterenol bitartrate) 4 mcg per min.
Available: Levophed 2 mg in 500 cc NS.
Administration set: microdrop.

   a. What is the rate of infusion in cc/min?

   b. What is the drop rate?

41. Order: Chloromycetin® (chloramphenicol sodium) 1 Gm IVPB q6h. Administer over 45 minutes.
    Available: Chloromycetin 1 Gm in 100 mL of D5W.
    Administration set: 20 gtts/mL.

    For how many gtts/min should you regulate the IV?

42. Order: Cefobid® (cefoperazone) 2 Gm IVPB q12h.
    Available: Cefobid 2 Gm in 50 mL NS to run at 100 cc/h.
    Administration set: 10 gtts/mL.

    a. For how many drops per minute should you regulate the IV?

    b. The IV was started at 2 p.m.; at this rate what time should the IV be completed?

43. Order: Heparin® (heparin sodium) 1000 U/hr continuous IV. Add 25,000 U Heparin to 1000 cc D5W.
    Administration set: microdrop.

    You should regulate the IV at how many gtts/min?

44. Order: Add 40 mEq KCl (potassium chloride) to 150 cc of D5W and administer at 8 mEq per hour.
    Administration set: microdrop.

    What should be the rate in gtts/min?

45. Order: Morphine sulfate 4 mg/hr IV by way of an electronic infusion device.
    Available: Morphine sulfate 50 mg/50 mL.

The infusion was started at 0700. At 1500 the infusion was discontinued.

a. How many mg of Morphine had the patient received?

b. How many mL of the original amount of the drug remain?

46. Order: Dopamine 2 µg/kg/min.
    Available: Dopamine 200 mg in 250 mL D5W.
    Patient's weight: 210 lbs.

    How fast would you regulate the IV on an electronic flow device?

47. A 50-mL piggyback is to infuse in 30 minutes.
    Administration set: 15 gtts/mL.
    Fifteen minutes after you started the infusion it contains 40 mL.

    Calculate the flow rate to deliver the medication on time.

48. Order: Amoxil® (amoxicillin) 200 mg in 50 mL D5W IVPB to infuse
            in 20 minutes q 6 hrs.
    Available: Electronic Regulating Device.

    How fast should you program the device?

49. Order: 250 mL D5W 1/2 NS IV with 20 mEq KCl to infuse at
            1 mEq/hr.
    Available: Buretrol Administration Set.

    What is the drip rate?

50. Order: Aminophylline® (theophylline ethylenediamine) IV at
    1 mg/kg/hr.
    Available: Aminophylline 250 mg in 500 cc D5W.
    Administration set: 15 gtts/mL.
    Patient's weight: 70 kg.

    You should regulate the IV at how many drops per minute?

51. Order: 2500 cc NS IV to infuse at 125 mL/hr.
    Administration set: 20 gtts/mL.

    a. How long will it take to infuse at this rate?

    b. IV was started at 0700. When will it be completed?

    c. What is the flow rate?

52. Order: 500 mL D5RL IV at 125 mL/hr. Was started at 1530; at 1730
    you notice 180 mL remaining.
    Administration set: 15 gtts/mL.

    a. How many mL should have infused by 1730?

    b. Regulate the IV to be completed on the original time schedule.

53. Your IV is infusing at 25 mL/h.
    Available: Heparin sodium 20,000 U in 500 mL D5W.

    How many units per hour is the patient receiving?

54. Calculate the infusion time for an IV of 1000 mL NS running at 25 gtts/min.
Administration set: 10 gtts/mL.

55. The flow rate on the IV is 22 gtts/min. 750 mL of D5RL remain to infuse.
Administration set: 20 gtts/mL.

At this rate, how long will it take to infuse?

56. 370 mL remain in the IV bag. The drip rate is 33 gtts/min, with a 15 gtts/mL administration set. It is 1300 hours. At what time will the infusion be completed?

57. It is 1400 hours and the IV is dripping at 54 gtts/min. 800 mL remain in the IV bag.
Administration set: 20 gtts/mL.

a. At this rate, how long will it take the IV to infuse?

b. At what hour will it be completed?

58. Order: Isuprel® (isoproterenol) 40 mL/hr IV.
Available: Isuprel 2 mg in 500 mL D5W.

How many mcg/min is the patient receiving?

59. Order: Nipride® (nitroprusside sodium) 6 mcg/kg/min IV.
Available: Nipride 50 mg in 250 mL D5W.
Administration set: 20 gtts/mL.
Patient's weight: 165 lbs.

At how many gtts per minute should you regulate the IV?

60. Order: Prostaphlin® (oxacillin sodium) 1-Gm IV push q.4.h.
    Available: Prostaphlin 2-Gm vial of powdered medication. Directions:
                Add 5 mL of Sterile Water for Injection to the 250-mg and
                500-mg vial; 10 mL to the 1-Gm vial and 20 mL to the
                2-Gm vial; and 40 mL to the 4-Gm vial.
    Rate of administration: 10 minutes

    a. How much diluent should you add?

    b. How many mL should you administer over 10 min _____ , 1 min
       _____ , 30 sec _____ , and 15 sec _____ ?

61. Order: Lanoxin® (digoxin) 150 μg IV push STAT via Heparin lock.
    Available: Lanoxin 0.5 mg/2-mL ampule. The literature recommends
                that Lanoxin should be diluted with a fourfold or greater
                volume of Sterile Water for Injection or 0.9% Sodium Chlo-
                ride for administration over 5 minutes or longer.

    a. How many mg are equal to 150 μg?

    b. How many milliliters of Lanoxin (0.5 mg/2 mL) should you prepare
       for administration?

    c. You would add the Lanoxin you prepared to how many milliliters
       of diluent?

    d. How many milliliters of Lanoxin and diluent are contained in the
       syringe?

    e. If you administered the total volume over 6 minutes, what portion
       of a mL would you give every 15 seconds?

62. Order: Velban® (vinblastine sulfate) 7.4 mg/M² IV push once a week.
    Patient's M² = 1.6 (125 lbs).
    Available: Velban 10 mg, 10-mL size vial—dry powder. Add 10 mL
           of Sodium Chloride for Injection to prepare a 1 mg/mL
           solution.
    Rate of administration: over 1 minute.

    a. How many mg of Velban should you administer?

    b. How many mL will you administer over 1 minute _____ , 30 seconds _____ , and 15 seconds _____ ?

    c. How many vials would you reconstitute?

Infants and Children

63. The recommended digitalizing dose of Digoxin® (lanoxin) for a child
    under 2 years is 35 μg/kg.
    Child's weight: 21 lbs.
    Available: Digoxin Elixir 0.05 mg/mL.

    How many mL should you administer?

64. Order: Versed® (midazolam hydrochloride) 4 mg IM on call.
    Child's weight: 30 kg.
    The manufacturer recommends 0.08–0.2 mg/kg dose q8h.

    Is the dose prescribed within the safe dose range?

65. An infant weighed 8 lbs 8 oz. The physician ordered Tagamet® (cimetidine) 20 mg/kg/day p.o. divided into 4 equal doses.
    Available: Tagamet Syrup 150 mg/5 mL.

    How many mL should you administer per dose?

66. Order: Phenergan® (promethazine hydrochloride) 1 mg/kg IM on call OR.
    Available: Phenergan ampule 25 mg/mL.
    Child's weight: 45 lbs.

    How many mL would you give?

    Use the following formula:

    $$\frac{(\text{Four times child's weight in kg}) + 7}{(\text{Child's weight in kg}) + 90} = \text{BSA}$$

67. Order: Benadryl Elixir® (diphenhydramine hydrochloride)
    150 mg/m²/day in 4 evenly divided doses.
    Available: Benadryl Elixir 12.5 mg/5 mL.
    Child's weight: 37 kg.

    How many mL should you administer per dose?

68. The recommended dose of Thorazine® (chlorpromazine) for a child is 60 mg/m²/24 h.
    Available: Thorazine Syrup 30 mg/5 mL.
    Child's weight: 60 lbs.

    How many mL should you administer q6h?

69. Order: Ilosone® (erythromycin estolate) 250 mg po qid.
    Available: Ilosone suspension 125 mg/5 mL.
    Child's weight: 33 lbs.
    Recommended dose: 50 mg/kg/day po in 2 equally divided doses q 12 h.

    What should you do about this order?

70. Order: Ceclor® (cefaclor) 325 mg q8h.
    Child's weight: 36 kg.
    Recommended dose: 20 to 40 mg/kg/day in divided doses every 8–12
    hours. Maximum dose 1 g/day.

    a. What is the minimum and maximum dose?

    b. Is the prescribed dose safe?

71. Order: Kantrex® (kanamycin sulfate) 50 mg BID IV in 100 mL D5W
    over 1 hour.
    Available: Kantrex 75 mg/2 mL.
    Recommended dose: Kantrex 15 mg/kg/day given in 2 equally divided
    doses.
    Child's weight: 11 lbs.

    Is the ordered dose safe? What should you do?

72. Ordered: Ancef® (cefazolin sodium) 300 mg IM q6h.
    Recommended dose: 25–50 mg/kg/day divided into four equal doses.
    Child's weight: 44 lbs.

    Is the prescribed dose safe?

73. Order: Phenobarbital 15 mg p.o. BID.
    Available: Phenobarbital 20 mg/5 mL oral suspension.
    Child's weight: 4.5 kg.
    Recommended dose: 5–7 mg/kg/day.

    Is the ordered dose safe?

74. Order: V-Cillin K® (penicillin V potassium) 250 mg po q8h.
    Available: V-Cillin K oral suspension 125 mg/5 mL.

Recommended dose: 25–50 mg/kg/day.
Child's weight: 45 lbs.

Is the ordered dose safe? What should you do?

75. Order: Bactopen® (cloxacillin sodium) 100 mg po qid.
Available: Bactopen 125 mg/5 mL oral solution.
Recommended dose: 50–100 mg/kg/day in equally divided doses every
6 hours.
Child's weight: 19 lbs.

a. Is the prescribed dose safe?

b. How much would you administer to equal one dose?

☐ Answers

Interpretation of Labels

1. a. Clinoril®
   b. Sulindac, MSD
   c. Tablet
   d. 200 mg/tablet
   e. 60
   f. Merck Sharp & Dohme
2. a. Synthroid®
   b. Levothyroxine sodium
   c. 200 mcg
   d. IV
   e. 0.9% Sodium Chloride Injection; Bacteriostatic Sodium Chloride
      Injection with Benzyl Alcohol
   f. 5 mL
   g. Use immediately—unused portion should be discarded
3. a. DHT™
   b. Dihydrotachysterol
   c. Tablets
   d. 0.125 mg/tablet
   e. 50
   f. Roxane

Calculation of Equivalents

4. 1 Gm : 1000 mg :: 0.080 Gm : X mg

$$1 X = 80 \text{ mg}$$

5. ½ oz : 4 dr :: ¾ oz : X dr

$$\tfrac{1}{2} X = {}^{12}\!/_4$$

$$X = 6 \text{ dr } (\text{z vi})$$

6. 1 gr : 60 mg :: ¹⁄₁₀₀ gr : X mg

$$1 X = {}^{60}\!/_{100}$$

$$X = 0.6 \text{ mg}$$

(if equivalent 15 gr : 1000 mg, X = 0.66 mg)

7. 1 tsp : 4 mL :: ⅛ tsp : X mL

$$1 X = \tfrac{4}{8} \text{ mL } (0.5 \text{ mL})$$

1 mL : 16 ℳ :: 0.5 mL : X ℳ

$$1 X = 8 \text{ ℳ } (\text{ℳ viii})$$

8. 1 mg : 1000 μg :: 6.5 mg : X μg

$$1 X = 6500 \text{ μg}$$

9. 1 glass : 8 oz :: 2½ glasses : X oz

$$1 X = 20 \text{ oz}$$

1 oz : 30 mL :: 20 oz : X mL

$$1 X = 600 \text{ mL}$$

10. 2.2 lbs : 1 kg :: 33 lbs : X kg

$$2.2 X = 33$$

$$X = 15 \text{ kg}$$

11. 1 tbsp : ½ oz :: 5½ tbsp : X oz

$$1 X = 2\tfrac{3}{4} \text{ oz}$$

12. 0.06 Gm : 1 gr :: 0.02 Gm : X gr

$$0.06 X = 0.02$$

$$X = 0.333 \text{ gr}$$

(if equivalent 1 Gm : 15 gr, X = ³⁄₁₀ gr or ⅓ gr)

13. 1 mL : 16 ℳ :: 0.45 mL : X ℳ

      1 X = 7.2 ℳ or 7 ℳ (ℳ vii)

14. 1 mg : $\frac{1}{60}$ gr :: 300 mg : X gr

      1 X = $\frac{300}{60}$ = 5 gr (gr v)

  (if equivalent 1000 mg : 15 gr, X = 4.5 gr (gr ivss)

15. 1 tsp : 5 mL :: 3⅓ tsp : X mL

      1 X = 16.6 mL

16. 1000 mg : 1 Gm :: 1750 mg : X Gm

      1000 X = 1750

          X = 1.75 Gm

17. 1 dr : 4 mL :: 4.2 dr : X mL

      1 X = 16.8 mL

18. 1 gr : 0.06 Gm :: 4 gr : X Gm

      1 X = 0.24 Gm

  (if equivalent 15 gr : 1 Gm, X = 0.266 Gm)

Oral Medications

19. a. 125 mg : 5 mL :: 500 mg : X mL

        125 X = 2500

           X = 20 mL

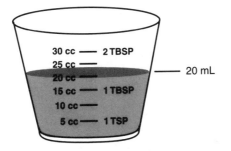

FIGURE 12.32.

  b. 2100

20. a. 1 Gm : 1000 mg :: 1.5 Gm : X mg

$$1 X = 1500 \text{ mg}$$

750 mg : 1 tab :: 1500 mg : X tab

$$750 X = 1500$$

$$X = 2 \text{ tabs}$$

b. It is yellow, oval and has the ⊜ symbol and K-Tab imprinted on the tablet.

c. 20 mEq

21. 1000 mg : 1 g :: X mg : 0.1 g

$$1 X = 100 \text{ mg}$$

5 ml = 1 tsp

50 mg : 1 tsp :: 100 mg : X tsp

$$50 X = 100$$

$$X = 2 \text{ tsp}$$

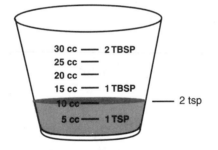

FIGURE 12.33.

22. a. 1 gr : 60 mg :: ⅓ gr : X mg

$$1 X = {}^{60}\!/_{3} = 20 \text{ mg}$$

10 mg : 1 tab :: 20 mg : X tab

$$10 X = 20$$

$$X = 2 \text{ tablets}$$

b. 2.2 lbs : 1 kg :: 121 lbs : X kg

$$2.2 X = 121$$

$$X = 55 \text{ kg}$$

0.4 mg : 1 kg :: X mg : 55 kg

1 X = 22 mg

0.8 mg : 1 kg :: X mg : 55 kg

1 X = 44 mg

Patient receiving 40 mg per day, which is within the recommended range.

23. 1000 mcg : 1 mg :: 750 mcg : X mg

1000 X = 750

X = 0.750 mg

0.375 mg : 1 tablet :: 0.750 mg : X tab

0.375 X = 0.750

X = 2 tablets

Parenteral Medications

24.

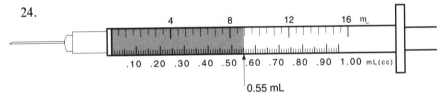

FIGURE 12.34.

1000 mcg : 1 mg :: 550 mcg : X mg

1000 X = 550

X = 0.55 mg

1 mg : mL :: 0.55 mg : X mL

1 X = 0.55 mL

25. a. 10 mg : 1 mL :: 25 mg : X mL

10 X = 25

X = 2.5 mL

b. 40 mg

c. Single-dose vial

d. IM or IV

26. 1 mg : $\frac{1}{60}$ gr :: 5 mg : X gr

$$1 X = \frac{5}{60} \text{ or } \frac{1}{12} \text{ gr}$$

$$\frac{1}{12} \text{ gr} : 16 \, \text{\textmu} :: \frac{1}{20} \text{ gr} : X \, \text{\textmu}$$

$$\frac{1}{12} X = \frac{16}{20}$$

$$X = 9.6 \, \text{\textmu} \text{ or } 10 \, \text{\textmu}$$

(If you measured in a 1-cc tuberculin syringe, you could measure 9.5 minims and add just a fraction to estimate the 0.1 to equal 9.6 minims. But if you were using a 3-cc syringe, you would have to round to 10 to get closest to the dose. The TB syringe would give you the closest dose.)

27. a. 2.2 lbs : 1 kg :: 99 lbs : X kg

$$2.2 X = 99$$

$$X = 45 \text{ kg}$$

$$5 \, \text{\textmu g} : 1 \text{ kg} :: X \, \text{\textmu g} : 45 \text{ kg}$$

$$1 X = 225 \, \text{\textmu g}$$

b. 1 mg : 1000 μg :: 0.5 mg : X μg

$$1 X = 500 \, \text{\textmu g}$$

$$500 \, \text{\textmu g} : 1 \text{ mL} :: 225 \, \text{\textmu g} : X \text{ mL}$$

$$500 X = 225$$

$$X = 0.45 \text{ mL}$$

28. a. 30 mg : 1 mL :: 25 mg : X mL

$$30 X = 25$$

$$X = 0.83 \text{ or } 0.8 \text{ mL}$$

b. 0.2 mL

Reconstitution of Powders and Crystals

29. a. 3.6 mL

b. 250 mg : 1 mL :: 750 mg : X mL

$$250 X = 750$$

$$X = 3 \text{ mL}$$

30. Use two vials of Desferal. Add 2 mL of Sterile Water for Injection to each vial. Withdraw the total volume (2 mL) from one vial and 1

mL from the second vial to obtain a total of 3 mL, which equals 750 mg.

$$250 \text{ mg} : 1 \text{ mL} :: 750 \text{ mg} : X \text{ mL}$$

$$250 \text{ X} = 750$$

$$X = 3 \text{ mL}$$

31. a. 6.8 mL

    b. $2000 \text{ mg} : 8 \text{ mL} :: 500 \text{ mg} : X \text{ mL}$

$$2000 \text{ X} = 4000$$

$$X = 2 \text{ mL}$$

    c.   8.0 mL TRV
       −6.8 mL Solvent
         1:2 mL Displacement

    d. June 5 at 6 a.m.

Insulin

32. a.

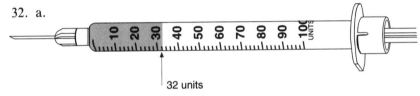

32 units

FIGURE 12.35.

    b. Tuberculin syringe

    c. $100 \text{ U} : 1 \text{ mL} :: 32 \text{ U} : X \text{ mL}$

$$100 \text{ X} = 32$$

$$X = 0.32 \text{ mL}$$

33. A blood sugar of 275 would require 13 units of insulin. The Lo-Dose syringe allows for a more precise measurement, because it has single units and the U-100 1 cc is measured in increments of 2.

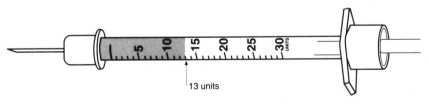

13 units

FIGURE 12.36.

34. a. Novolin L 25 units + 6 units Novolin R = 31 units

    b. Novolin L = 25 + 18 = 43
       Novolin R = 6 + 8 = $\underline{14}$
       Total   57

35. a. 49 units

    b. U-100 1 cc syringe

    c. Tuberculin syringe

    d. Humulin N = 0.42 mL
       Humulin R = $\underline{0.07\ mL}$
                    0.49 mL

Intravenous Fluids and Medications

36. $\dfrac{500\ cc}{12\ hours} \times \dfrac{15\ gtts/mL}{60\ minutes} = 10.4$ or 10 gtts/min

37. $\dfrac{75\ cc}{60\ minutes} \times 10\ gtts/mL = 13$ gtts/min

38. a. $\dfrac{1000\ cc}{6\ hours} \times \dfrac{20\ gtts/mL}{60\ minutes} = 55.5$ or 56 gtts/min

    b. 1000 cc ÷ 6 hours = 167 cc per hour × 4 hours = 668 cc

    c. $\dfrac{450\ cc}{2\ hours} \times \dfrac{20\ gtts/mL}{60\ minutes} = 75$ gtts/min

39. a. 15 gtts : 1 mL :: 26 gtts : X mL

              15 X = 26

                 X = 1.73 cc per minute

    b. 1.7 cc : 1 minute :: 450 cc : X minutes

              1.7 X = 450

                  X = 265 minutes

       60 minutes : 1 hour :: 265 minutes : X hours

              60 X = 265

                 X = 4.4 hours, or 4 hours 24 minutes

40. 2 mg = 2000 μg

    a. 2000 μg : 500 cc :: 4 μg : X cc

$$2000 \ X \ = \ 2000$$

$$X \ = \ 1 \ cc/min$$

    b. 1 cc per minute × 60 gtts/cc = 60 gtts/min

41. $\dfrac{100 \ mL}{45 \ minutes}$ × 20 gtts/mL = 44.4 or 44 gtts/min

42. a. $\dfrac{100 \ cc}{60 \ minutes}$ × 10 gtts/cc = 16.6 or 17 gtts/min

    b. 100 cc : 60 minutes :: 50 cc : X minutes

$$100 \ X \ = \ 3000$$

$$X \ = \ 30 \ minutes \ or \ 2:30 \ p.m.$$

43. 25,000 U : 1000 cc :: 1000 U : X cc

$$25,000 \ X \ = \ 1,000,000$$

$$X \ = \ 40 \ cc$$

$\dfrac{40 \ cc}{60 \ minutes}$ × 60 gtts/cc = 40 gtts/min

44. 40 mEq : 150 cc :: 8 mEq : X cc

$$40 \ X \ = \ 1200$$

$$X \ = \ 30 \ cc$$

$\dfrac{30 \ cc}{60 \ minutes}$ × 60 gtts/cc = 30 gtts/min

45. a. Between 0700 and 1500 = 8 hours @ 4 mg = 32 mg

    b. 32 mg = 32 mL

$$50 \ mL \ - \ 32 \ mL \ = \ 18 \ mL \ remain$$

46. 210 lbs = 95.5 or 96 kg

2 mcg × 96 kg = 192 mcg/min × 60 min = 11,520 mcg/h

200,000 mcg : 250 mL :: 11,520 mcg : X mL

$$200,000 \ X \ = \ 2,880,000$$

$$X \ = \ 14.4 \ or \ 14 \ cc/h$$

47. $\dfrac{40 \text{ mL}}{15 \text{ min}} \times 15 \text{ gtts/mL} = 40 \text{ gtts/min}$

48. 50 mL : 20 minutes :: X mL : 60 minutes

$$20 \text{ X} = 3000$$

$$\text{X} = 150 \text{ mL/h}$$

49. 250 mL : 20 mEq :: X mL : 1 mEq

$$20 \text{ X} = 250$$

$$\text{X} = 12.5 \text{ mL/h}$$

$\dfrac{12.5 \text{ mL}}{1 \text{ hour}} \times \dfrac{60 \text{ gtts/mL}}{60 \text{ minutes}} = 12.5 \text{ gtts/min}$

50. 1 mg × 70 kg = 70 mg/h

70 mg : X mL :: 250 mg : 500 mL

$$250 \text{ X} = 35,000$$

$$\text{X} = 140 \text{ mL/h}$$

$\dfrac{140 \text{ mL}}{1 \text{ hour}} \times \dfrac{15 \text{ gtts/mL}}{60 \text{ minutes}} = 35 \text{ gtts/min}$

51. a. 2500 cc : X hours :: 125 cc : 1 hour

$$125 \text{ X} = 2500$$

$$\text{X} = 20 \text{ hours}$$

    b. 0300

    c. $\dfrac{125 \text{ cc}}{1 \text{ hour}} \times \dfrac{20 \text{ gtts/mL}}{60 \text{ minutes}} = 41.6 \text{ or } 42 \text{ gtts/min}$

52. a. 2 hours × 125 mL = 250 mL by 1730

    b. $\dfrac{180 \text{ mL}}{2 \text{ hours}} \times \dfrac{15 \text{ gtts/mL}}{60 \text{ minutes}} = 22.5 \text{ or } 23 \text{ gtts/min}$

53. 20,000 U : 500 mL :: X U : 25 mL

$$500 \text{ X} = 500,000$$

$$\text{X} = 1000 \text{ U/h}$$

54. $\text{X} = \dfrac{1000 \text{ mL}}{25 \text{ gtts}} \times \dfrac{10 \text{ gtts/mL}}{60 \text{ minutes}} = \begin{array}{l} 6.66 \text{ or } 6 \text{ hours and } 40 \text{ minutes} \\ (6.7 = 6 \text{ hours and } 42 \text{ minutes}) \end{array}$

55. $\text{X} = \dfrac{750 \text{ mL}}{22 \text{ gtts}} \times \dfrac{20 \text{ gtts/mL}}{60 \text{ minutes}} = \begin{array}{l} 11.36 \text{ or } 11 \text{ hours and } 22 \text{ minutes} \\ (11.4 = 11 \text{ hours and } 24 \text{ minutes}) \end{array}$

56. $$X = \frac{250 \text{ mL}}{33 \text{ gtts}} \times \frac{15 \text{ gtts/mL}}{60 \text{ minutes}} = \begin{array}{l} 1.89 \text{ or } 1 \text{ hour and } 53 \text{ minutes} \\ (1.9 = 1 \text{ hour and } 54 \text{ minutes}) \end{array}$$

The IV should have been completed at approximately 1454 hours.

57. a. 54 gtts : X mL : : 20 gtts/mL : 1 mL

$$20 \text{ X} = 54$$

$$X = 2.7 \text{ mL/min} \times 60 \text{ minutes} = 162 \text{ mL/h}$$

800 mL : X hours : : 162 mL : 1 hour

$$162 \text{ X} = 800$$

$$X = 4.9 \text{ or } 4 \text{ hours and } 54 \text{ minutes}$$

   b. IV completed at approximately 1854

58. 2000 mcg : 500 mL : : X mcg : 40 mL

$$500 \text{ X} = 80,000$$

$$X = 160 \text{ mcg/h} \div 60 \text{ minutes}$$

$$= 2.66 \text{ or } 2.7 \text{ mcg/min}$$

59. 165 lbs = 75 kg

   6 mcg × 75 kg = 450 mcg/min

   50 mg = 50,000 mcg

   50,000 mcg : 250 mL : : 450 mcg : X mL

$$50,000 \text{ X} = 112,500$$

$$X = 2.25 \text{ mL/min}$$

   2.3 mL/min × 20 gtts/mL = 46 gtts/min

60. a. 20 mL

   b. 2 Gm : 20 mL : : 1 Gm : X mL

$$2 \text{ X} = 20$$

$$X = 10 \text{ mL equal the dosage}$$

   10 minutes = 10 mL

   1 minute = 1 mL

   30 seconds = 0.5 mL

   15 seconds = 0.25 mL

61. a. 1 mg : 1000 μg :: X mg : 150 μg

$$1000\ X\ =\ 150$$

$$X\ =\ 0.15\ mg$$

   b. 0.5 mg : 2 mL :: 0.15 mg : X mL

$$0.5\ X\ =\ 0.3$$

$$X\ =\ 0.6\ mL$$

   c.   0.6 mL Lanoxin
$$\underline{\times\ 4\ (\text{4-fold the dosage volume})}$$
2.4 mL Diluent

   d.   2.4 mL Diluent
$$\underline{+\,0.6\ mL\ Lanoxin}$$
3.0 mL Total fluid

   e. 3 mL : 360 seconds :: X mL : 15 seconds

$$360\ X\ =\ 45$$

$$X\ =\ 0.125\ mL\ per\ 15\ seconds$$

62. a. 7.4 mg : 1 m² :: X mg : 1.6 m²

$$1\ X\ =\ 11.84\ mg$$

   b. 10 mg : 10 ml :: 11.84 mg : X mL

$$10\ X\ =\ 118.4$$

$$X\ =\ 11.84\ mL\ over\ 1\ minute$$

   5.9 or 6 mL in 30 seconds

   2.9 or 3 mL in 15 seconds

   c. 2 vials

Infants and Children

63. 21 lbs = 9.54 kg

$$35\ μg\ \times\ 9.54\ kg\ =\ 333.9\ μg$$

$$1\ mg:\ 1000\ μg\ ::\ X\ mg\ :\ 333.9\ μg$$

$$1000\ X\ =\ 333.9$$

$$X\ =\ 0.334\ mg$$

$$0.05\ mg\ :\ 1\ mL\ ::\ 0.334\ mg\ :\ X\ mL$$

$$0.05\ X\ =\ 0.334$$

$$X\ =\ 6.68\ or\ 6.7\ cc$$

64. 0.05 mg/kg

$$0.08 \text{ mg} \times 30 \text{ kg} = 2.4 \text{ mg}$$

0.2 mg/kg

$$0.2 \text{ mg} \times 30 \text{ kg} = 6 \text{ mg}$$

Dose of 4 mg is within the safe range.

65. 8.5 lbs = 3.86 kg

$$20 \text{ mg} \times 3.86 \text{ kg} = 77.2 \text{ mg} \div 4 \text{ doses} = 19.3 \text{ mg/dose}$$

$$150 \text{ mg} : 5 \text{ mL} :: 19.3 \text{ mg} : X \text{ mL}$$

$$150 \text{ X} = 96.5$$

$$X = 0.64 \text{ mL q6h}$$

66. 45 lbs = 20.45 kg

$$1 \text{ mg} \times 20.45 \text{ kg} = 20.45 \text{ mg}$$

$$25 \text{ mg} : 1 \text{ mL} :: 20.45 \text{ mg} : X \text{ mL}$$

$$25 \text{ X} = 20.45$$

$$X = 0.818 \text{ or } 0.82 \text{ mL}$$

67. BSA

$$\frac{(4 \times 37) + 7}{37 + 90} = \frac{155}{127} = 1.22 \text{ BSA m}^2$$

$$150 \text{ mg} \times 1.22 \text{ BSA} = 183 \text{ mg/day} \div 4 \text{ doses} = 45.75 \text{ mg/dose}$$

$$12.5 \text{ mg} : 5 \text{ mL} :: 45.75 \text{ mg} : X \text{ mL}$$

$$12.5 \text{ X} = 228.75$$

$$X = 18.3 \text{ or } 18 \text{ mL per dose}$$

68. 60 lbs = 27.27 kg

BSA

$$\frac{(4 \times 27.27) + 7}{27.27 + 90} = \frac{116.08}{117.27} = 0.98985 \text{ BSA m}^2 = 0.990$$

$$0.990 \text{ BSA} \times 60 \text{ mg} = 59.4 \text{ mg/24 hours}$$

$$59.4 \text{ mg} \div 4 \text{ (q6h)} = 14.85 \text{ mg per dose}$$

$$30 \text{ mg} : 5 \text{ mL} :: 14.85 \text{ mg} : X \text{ mL}$$

$$30 \text{ X} = 74.25$$

$$X = 2.475 \text{ or } 2.5 \text{ mL}$$

69. 33 lbs = 15 kg

15 kg × 50 mg = 750 mg/day ÷ 2 = 375 mg/dose

The individual dose of 250 mg is within the recommended amount, but the total for the day according to the order would be 250 mg × 4 (qid) = 1000 mg, or 250 mg more than the total recommended dose. Notify the physician before proceeding.

70. a. Minimum dose = 36 kg × 20 mg = 720 mg
      (q8h = 240-mg dose; q12h = 360-mg dose)

   Maximum dose = 36 kg × 40 mg = 1440 mg
      (q8h = 480-mg dose; q12hr = 720-mg dose)

   b. The dose is safe. 350 mg is within the 240–480 mg range per dose for a q8h schedule.

71. 11 lbs = 5 kg

5 kg × 15 mg = 75 mg ÷ 2 = 37.5 mg per dose

The ordered dose is not a safe dose. You should notify the physician.

72. 44 lbs = 20 kg

20 kg × 25 mg = 500 mg ÷ 4 = 125 mg per dose

20 kg × 50 mg = 1000 mg ÷ 4 = 250 mg per dose

The prescribed dose exceeds the recommended dose. Notify the physician.

73. The ordered dose is at the upper limits of the recommended range. The total dose ordered would be 30 mg per day.

5 mg × 4.5 kg = 22.5 mg per day

7 mg × 4.5 kg = 31.5 mg per day

Administer the drug.

$$20 \text{ mg} : 5 \text{ mL} :: 15 \text{ mg} : X \text{ mL}$$

$$20 X = 75$$

$$X = 3.75 \text{ mL}$$

74. The prescribed dose of 250 mg/dose or 750 mg/day is within the recommended dose.

45 lbs = 20.5 kg

25 mg × 20.5 kg = 512.5 mg/day

50 mg × 20.5 kg = 1025 mg/day

Administer 10 mL each dose.

$$250 \text{ mg} : X \text{ mL} :: 125 \text{ mg} : 5 \text{ mL}$$

$$125 \text{ X} = 1250$$

$$X = 10 \text{ mL}$$

75. a. The prescribed dose of 100 mg per dose or 400 mg/day is a safe dose. It is slightly under the recommended dose, and you might mention this to the physician.

19 lbs = 8.6 kg

50 mg $\times$ 8.6 kg = 430 mg $\div$ 4 = 107.5 mg per dose

100 mg $\times$ 8.6 kg = 860 mg $\div$ 4 = 215 mg per dose

b. 125 mg : 5 mL :: 100 mg : X mL

$$125 \text{ X} = 500$$

$$X = 4 \text{ mL per dose}$$

Appendix

Temperature Conversion

It may be necessary to convert Fahrenheit temperatures to Celsius (centigrade) and vice versa. To do so, use the following conversion formulas:

Fahrenheit to Celsius

$$C = \frac{5 \times \text{``F''} - 160}{9}$$

Celsius to Fahrenheit

$$F = \frac{9 \times \text{``C''} + 160}{5}$$

Follow these steps when using either formula:

1. Multiply the temperature by 5 or 9.

2. Add or subtract 160.

3. Divide by 9 or 5.

It is important that the steps are done in this order.

Example

a. 98.6° F = ? Celsius

$$C = \frac{5 \times 98.6 - 160}{9}$$

$$= \frac{493 - 160}{9}$$

$$= \frac{333}{9}$$

$$= 37° \text{ Celsius}$$

b. 32° C = ? Fahrenheit

$$F = \frac{9 \times 32 + 160}{5}$$

$$= \frac{288 + 160}{5}$$

$$= \frac{448}{5}$$

$$= 89.6° \text{ Fahrenheit}$$

☐ Practice Problems

Complete the following conversions:

	Fahrenheit	Celsius
1.	101°	____
2.	____	38.9°
3.	100°	____
4.	____	10°
5.	95°	____
6.	____	50°

☐ Answers

	Fahrenheit	Celsius
1.	101°	38.3°
2.	102°	38.9°
3.	100°	37.8°
4.	50°	10°
5.	95°	35°
6.	122°	50°

Military Time

Many hospitals and health care agencies use "military time" as the basis for their time-keeping system. Military time is a 24-hour system that uses digital numbers to indicate morning, afternoon, and evening times. Military time is based on 100 increments of time, beginning with 0100, which is the equivalent of 1:00 AM. Each additional hour is increased by 100 until 2400 hours or midnight.

Comparison of Times

Standard Clock Time	Military Time
12:30 AM	0030
1:00 AM	0100
2:00 AM	0200
6:00 AM	0600
7:30 AM	0730
Noon	1200
4:30 PM	1630
5:00 PM	1700
9:00 PM	2100

As you have probably noted, from midnight to noon the standard clock time notation and the military time are very similar. For the AM hours 1 to 9, you would read them as 0100 (zero-100) or 1 AM until you reached 10 AM. At 10 AM you would read it as ten-hundred hours through 12 noon or 1200 hours. After 12 noon or 1200 hours, the easiest way to convert standard clock time to military time is to add the hour (in increments of 100) to 1200 (twelve hundred). Nine (PM) in the evening would be 900 added to 1200, thus 2100 (twenty-one-hundred) hours. You perform the process in reverse to convert military time to standard clock time. To change PM times such as 1500 to standard time, subtract 1200, which in this case leaves 300 (each hour is in increment of 100) or 3:00 PM. Remember, with standard clock time you start numbering again after 12 noon. Mastering military time takes a little practice, but with each hour having a unique number it can decrease medication errors.

The next challenge is to figure out the minutes. The minute increments are the same for standard clock and military time, 60 increments per hour. From midnight (2400) to 1 AM (0100) is expressed in minutes such as 0001, 0002, 0015, 0030, and 0050. For example, 7:30 AM would be written 0730, or zero-730; 2:25 PM would be written 1425 (1200 plus 225); and 12:30 AM would actually be 0030, zero-zero-thirty.

If you have difficulty converting from standard clock time to military time, many digital watches will display both times. You can also make yourself a card to help you with the conversion. An example of a 24-hour clock is presented below. The numbers on the inside represent the hours from

The 24-hour clock

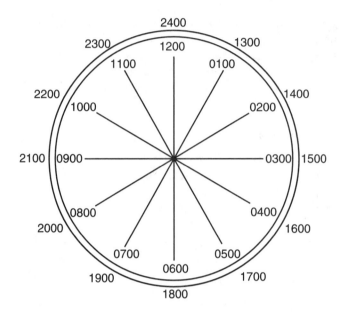

midnight to noon, and the outside numbers represent the time from noon until midnight.

☐ Practice Problems

Change the following times:

	Standard	*Military*
1.	4:00 PM	_____
2.	_____	0700
3.	_____	1530
4.	11:30 AM	_____
5.	9:00 PM	_____
6.	_____	2310
7.	12:15 AM	_____

8.   4:05 PM   ———

9.   2:00 AM   ———

10.   ———   0515

☐ **Answers**

1. 1600 (sixteen-hundred hours)
2. 7:00 AM
3. 3:30 PM
4. 1130 (eleven-thirty hours)
5. 2100 (twenty-one-hundred hours)
6. 11:10 PM
7. 0015 (zero-zero-fifteen hours)
8. 1605 (sixteen-zero-five hours)
9. 0200 (zero-two-hundred hours)
10. 5:15 AM

Credits

We appreciate the willingness of the pharmaceutical companies to grant us permission to use their drug labels and syringes. The companies who granted permission include:

Abbott Laboratories
AMGEN
Astra Pharmaceutical Products, Inc.
Becton Dickinson and Company
Boots Pharmaceuticals
Eli Lilly and Company
Medical Economics Data
Merck Sharp & Dohme
Miles Pharmaceutical Division
Novo Nordisk Pharmaceuticals Inc.
Roxane Laboratories, Inc.
Tap Pharmaceuticals Inc.
Terumo Medical Cooperation